BLACKWELL'S
UNDERGROUND CLINICAL VIGNETTES

BEHAVIORAL
SCIENCE, 3E

BLACKWELL'S
UNDERGROUND CLINICAL VIGNETTES

BEHAVIORAL SCIENCE, 3E

VIKAS BHUSHAN, MD
University of California, San Francisco, Class of 1991
Series Editor, Diagnostic Radiologist

VISHAL PALL, MBBS
Government Medical College, Chandigarh, India, Class of 1996
Series Editor, U. of Texas, Galveston, Resident in Internal Medicine &
Preventive Medicine

TAO LE, MD
University of California, San Francisco, Class of 1996

HOANG NGUYEN, MD, MBA
Northwestern University, Class of 2001

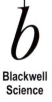

Blackwell
Science

CONTRIBUTORS

Ishnella Azad, MD
University of California Los Angeles, Resident in Psychiatry

Siddarth Shah, MD
Mt. Sinai School of Medicine, New York, Resident in Preventive
and Community Medicine

Fadi Abu Shahin, MD
University of Damascus, Syria, Class of 1999

Alexander Grimm, MD
St. Louis University School of Medicine, Class of 1999

Sunit Das, MD
Northwestern University, Class of 2000

FACULTY REVIEWER

Rita Joshi, MD
University of California Los Angeles, Attending Physician
in Psychiatry

© 2002 by Blackwell Science, Inc.

Editorial Offices:

Commerce Place, 350 Main Street, Malden,
    Massachusetts 02148, USA
Osney Mead, Oxford OX2 0EL, England
25 John Street, London WC1N 2BS, England
23 Ainslie Place, Edinburgh EH3 6AJ, Scotland
54 University Street, Carlton, Victoria 3053,
    Australia

Other Editorial Offices:

Blackwell Wissenschafts-Verlag GmbH,
    Kurfürstendamm 57, 10707 Berlin, Germany
Blackwell Science KK, MG Kodenmacho Building,
    7-10 Kodenmacho Nihombashi, Chuo-ku,
    Tokyo 104, Japan
Iowa State University Press, A Blackwell Science
    Company, 2121 S. State Avenue, Ames, Iowa
    50014-8300, USA

Distributors:

The Americas
Blackwell Publishing
c/o AIDC
P.O. Box 20
50 Winter Sport Lane
Williston, VT 05495-0020
(Telephone orders: 800-216-2522;
    fax orders: 802-864-7626)
Australia
Blackwell Science Pty, Ltd.
54 University Street
Carlton, Victoria 3053
(Telephone orders: 03-9347-0300;
    fax orders: 03-9349-3016)
Outside The Americas and Australia
Blackwell Science, Ltd.
c/o Marston Book Services, Ltd.
P.O. Box 269
Abingdon
Oxon OX14 4YN
England
(Telephone orders: 44-01235-465500;
    fax orders: 44-01235-465555)

Acquisitions: Laura DeYoung
Development: Amy Nuttbrock
Production: Lorna Hind and Shawn Girsberger
Manufacturing: Lisa Flanagan
Marketing Manager: Kathleen Mulcahy
Cover design by Leslie Haimes
Interior design by Shawn Girsberger
Typeset by TechBooks
Printed and bound by Capital City Press

Blackwell's Underground Clinical Vignettes:
    Behavioral Science, 3e
ISBN 0-632-04543-4

Printed in the United States of America
02 03 04 05 5 4 3 2 1

The Blackwell Science logo is a trade mark of
Blackwell Science Ltd., registered at the United
Kingdom Trade Marks Registry

Library of Congress Cataloging-in-Publication Data
Bhushan, Vikas.
Blackwell's underground clinical vignettes.
Behavioral science / author, Vikas Bhushan.– 3rd ed.
    p. ; cm. – (Underground clinical vignettes) Rev. ed.
of: Behavioral science / Vikas Bhushan ... [et al.].
2nd ed. c1998. ISBN 0-632-04543-4 (pbk.)
1. Psychiatry – Case studies. 2. Neuropsychiatry –
Case studies. 3. Behavioral sciences – Case studies.
4. Physicians – Licenses – United States –
Examinations – Study guides.
    [DNLM: 1. Behavioral Sciences – Case Report.
2. Behavioral Sciences – Problems and Exercises.
3. Mental Disorders – Case Report. 4. Mental
Disorders – Problems and Exercises. WM 18.2 B575ba
2002] I. Title: Underground clinical vignettes.
Behavioral science. II. Title: Behavioral science.
III. Behavioral science. IV. Title. V. Series.
    RC465 .B5259 2002
    616.89'0076–dc21

                                                    2001004886

CONTENTS

ACKNOWLEDGMENTS

Throughout the production of this book, we have had the support of many friends and colleagues. Special thanks to our support team including Anu Gupta, Andrea Fellows, Anastasia Anderson, Srishti Gupta, Mona Pall, Jonathan Kirsch and Chirag Amin. For prior contributions we thank Gianni Le Nguyen, Tarun Mathur, Alex Grimm, Sonia Santos and Elizabeth Sanders.

We have enjoyed working with a world-class international publishing group at Blackwell Science, including Laura DeYoung, Amy Nuttbrock, Lisa Flanagan, Shawn Girsberger, Lorna Hind and Gordon Tibbitts. For help with securing images for the entire series we also thank Lee Martin, Kristopher Jones, Tina Panizzi and Peter Anderson at the University of Alabama, the Armed Forces Institute of Pathology, and many of our fellow Blackwell Science authors.

For submitting comments, corrections, editing, proofreading, and assistance across all of the vignette titles in all editions, we collectively thank:

Tara Adamovich, Carolyn Alexander, Kris Alden, Henry E. Aryan, Lynman Bacolor, Natalie Barteneva, Dean Bartholomew, Debashish Behera, Sumit Bhatia, Sanjay Bindra, Dave Brinton, Julianne Brown, Alexander Brownie, Tamara Callahan, David Canes, Bryan Casey, Aaron Caughey, Hebert Chen, Jonathan Cheng, Arnold Cheung, Arnold Chin, Simion Chiosea, Yoon Cho, Samuel Chung, Gretchen Conant, Vladimir Coric, Christopher Cosgrove, Ronald Cowan, Karekin R. Cunningham, A. Sean Dalley, Rama Dandamudi, Sunit Das, Ryan Armando Dave, John David, Emmanuel de la Cruz, Robert DeMello, Navneet Dhillon, Sharmila Dissanaike, David Donson, Adolf Etchegaray, Alea Eusebio, Priscilla A. Frase, David Frenz, Kristin Gaumer, Yohannes Gebreegziabher, Anil Gehi, Tony George, L.M. Gotanco, Parul Goyal, Alex Grimm, Rajeev Gupta, Ahmad Halim, Sue Hall, David Hasselbacher, Tamra Heimert, Michelle Higley, Dan Hoit, Eric Jackson, Tim Jackson, Sundar Jayaraman, Pei-Ni Jone, Aarchan Joshi, Rajni K. Jutla, Faiyaz Kapadi, Seth Karp, Aaron S. Kesselheim, Sana Khan, Andrew Pin-wei Ko, Francis Kong, Paul Konitzky, Warren S. Krackov, Benjamin H.S. Lau, Ann LaCasce, Connie Lee, Scott Lee, Guillermo Lehmann, Kevin Leung, Paul Levett, Warren Levinson, Eric Ley, Ken Lin,

Pavel Lobanov, J. Mark Maddox, Aram Mardian, Samir Mehta, Gil Melmed, Joe Messina, Robert Mosca, Michael Murphy, Vivek Nandkarni, Siva Naraynan, Carvell Nguyen, Linh Nguyen, Deanna Nobleza, Craig Nodurft, George Noumi, Darin T. Okuda, Adam L. Palance, Paul Pamphrus, Jinha Park, Sonny Patel, Ricardo Pietrobon, Riva L. Rahl, Aashita Randeria, Rachan Reddy, Beatriu Reig, Marilou Reyes, Jeremy Richmon, Tai Roe, Rick Roller, Rajiv Roy, Diego Ruiz, Anthony Russell, Sanjay Sahgal, Urmimala Sarkar, John Schilling, Isabell Schmitt, Daren Schuhmacher, Sonal Shah, Fadi Abu Shahin, Mae Sheikh-Ali, Edie Shen, Justin Smith, John Stulak, Lillian Su, Julie Sundaram, Rita Suri, Seth Sweetser, Antonio Talayero, Merita Tan, Mark Tanaka, Eric Taylor, Jess Thompson, Indi Trehan, Raymond Turner, Okafo Uchenna, Eric Uyguanco, Richa Varma, John Wages, Alan Wang, Eunice Wang, Andy Weiss, Amy Williams, Brian Yang, Hany Zaky, Ashraf Zaman and David Zipf.

For generously contributing images to the entire *Underground Clinical Vignette* Step 1 series, we collectively thank the staff at Blackwell Science in Oxford, Boston, and Berlin as well as:

- Axford, J. *Medicine.* Osney Mead: Blackwell Science Ltd, 1996. Figures 2.14, 2.15, 2.16, 2.27, 2.28, 2.31, 2.35, 2.36, 2.38, 2.43, 2.65a, 2.65b, 2.65c, 2.103b, 2.105b, 3.20b, 3.21, 8.27, 8.27b, 8.77b, 8.77c, 10.81b, 10.96a, 12.28a, 14.6, 14.16, 14.50.

- Bannister B, Begg N, Gillespie S. *Infectious Disease, 2nd Edition.* Osney Mead: Blackwell Science Ltd, 2000. Figures 2.8, 3.4, 5.28, 18.10, W5.32, W5.6.

- Berg D. *Advanced Clinical Skills and Physical Diagnosis.* Blackwell Science Ltd., 1999. Figures 7.10, 7.12, 7.13, 7.2, 7.3, 7.7, 7.8, 7.9, 8.1, 8.2, 8.4, 8.5, 9.2, 10.2, 11.3, 11.5, 12.6.

- Cuschieri A, Hennessy TPJ, Greenhalgh RM, Rowley DA, Grace PA. *Clinical Surgery.* Osney Mead: Blackwell Science Ltd, 1996. Figures 13.19, 18.22, 18.33.

- Gillespie SH, Bamford K. *Medical Microbiology and Infection at a Glance.* Osney Mead: Blackwell Science Ltd, 2000. Figures 20, 23.

- Ginsberg L. *Lecture Notes on Neurology, 7th Edition.* Osney Mead: Blackwell Science Ltd, 1999. Figures 12.3, 18.3, 18.3b.

- Elliott T, Hastings M, Desselberger U. *Lecture Notes on Medical Microbiology, 3rd Edition.* Osney Mead: Blackwell Science Ltd, 1997. Figures 2, 5, 7, 8, 9, 11, 12, 14, 15, 16, 17, 19, 20, 25, 26, 27, 29, 30, 34, 35, 52.

- Mehta AB, Hoffbrand AV. *Haematology at a Glance.* Osney Mead: Blackwell Science Ltd, 2000. Figures 22.1, 22.2, 22.3.

Please let us know if your name has been missed or misspelled and we will be happy to make the update in the next edition.

PREFACE TO THE 3RD EDITION

We were very pleased with the overwhelmingly positive student feedback for the 2nd edition of our *Underground Clinical Vignettes* series. Well over 100,000 copies of the UCV books are in print and have been used by students all over the world.

Over the last two years we have accumulated and incorporated **over a thousand "updates"** and improvements suggested by you, our readers, including:

- many additions of specific boards and wards testable content

- deletions of redundant and overlapping cases

- reordering and reorganization of all cases in both series

- a new master index by case name in each Atlas

- correction of a few factual errors

- diagnosis and treatment updates

- addition of 5–20 new cases in every book

- and the addition of clinical exam photographs within *UCV—Anatomy*

And most important of all, the third edition sets now include two brand new **COLOR ATLAS** supplements, one for each Clinical Vignette series.

- The *UCV–Basic Science Color Atlas* (*Step 1*) includes over 250 color plates, divided into gross pathology, microscopic pathology (histology), hematology, and microbiology (smears).

- The *UCV–Clinical Science Color Atlas* (*Step 2*) has over 125 color plates, including patient images, dermatology, and funduscopy.

Each atlas image is descriptively captioned and linked to its corresponding Step 1 case, Step 2 case, and/or Step 2 MiniCase.

How Atlas Links Work:

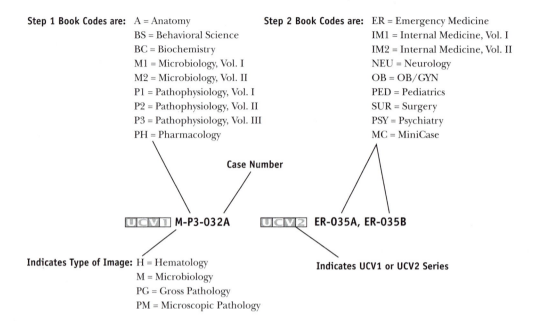

Step 1 Book Codes are:
A = Anatomy
BS = Behavioral Science
BC = Biochemistry
M1 = Microbiology, Vol. I
M2 = Microbiology, Vol. II
P1 = Pathophysiology, Vol. I
P2 = Pathophysiology, Vol. II
P3 = Pathophysiology, Vol. III
PH = Pharmacology

Step 2 Book Codes are:
ER = Emergency Medicine
IM1 = Internal Medicine, Vol. I
IM2 = Internal Medicine, Vol. II
NEU = Neurology
OB = OB/GYN
PED = Pediatrics
SUR = Surgery
PSY = Psychiatry
MC = MiniCase

Case Number

UCV1 M-P3-032A   UCV2 ER-035A, ER-035B

Indicates Type of Image:
H = Hematology
M = Microbiology
PG = Gross Pathology
PM = Microscopic Pathology

Indicates UCV1 or UCV2 Series

- If the Case number (032, 035, etc.) is not followed by a letter, then there is only one image. Otherwise A, B, C, D indicate up to 4 images.

Bold Faced Links: In order to give you access to the largest number of images possible, we have chosen to cross link the Step 1 and 2 series.

- If the link is bold-faced this indicates that the link is direct (i.e., Step 1 Case with the Basic Science Step 1 Atlas link).

- If the link is not bold-faced this indicates that the link is indirect (Step 1 case with Clinical Science Step 2 Atlas link or vice versa).

We have also implemented a few structural changes upon your request:

- Each current and future edition of our popular *First Aid for the USMLE Step 1* (Appleton & Lange/McGraw-Hill) and *First Aid for the USMLE Step 2* (Appleton & Lange/McGraw-Hill) book will be linked to the corresponding UCV case.

- We eliminated UCV → First Aid links as they frequently become out of date, as the *First Aid* books are revised yearly.

- The Color Atlas is also specially designed for quizzing—captions are descriptive and do not give away the case name directly.

We hope the updated UCV series will remain a unique and well-integrated study tool that provides compact clinical correlations to basic science information. They are designed to be easy and fun (comparatively) to read, and helpful for both licensing exams and the wards.

We invite your corrections and suggestions for the fourth edition of these books. For the first submission of each factual correction or new vignette that is selected for inclusion in the fourth edition, you will receive a personal acknowledgment in the revised book. If you submit over 20 high-quality corrections, additions or new vignettes we will also consider **inviting you to become a "Contributor" on the book of your choice**. If you are interested in becoming a potential "Contributor" or "Author" on a future UCV book, or working with our team in developing additional books, please also e-mail us your CV/resume.

We prefer that you submit corrections or suggestions via electronic mail to **UCVteam@yahoo.com**. Please include "Underground Vignettes" as the subject of your message. If you do not have access to e-mail, use the following mailing address: Blackwell Publishing, Attn: UCV Editors, 350 Main Street, Malden, MA 02148, USA.

Vikas Bhushan
Vishal Pall
Tao Le
October 2001

HOW TO USE THIS BOOK

This series was originally developed to address the increasing number of clinical vignette questions on medical examinations, including the USMLE Step 1 and Step 2. It is also designed to supplement and complement the popular *First Aid for the USMLE Step 1* (Appleton & Lange/McGraw Hill) and *First Aid for the USMLE Step 2* (Appleton & Lange/McGraw Hill).

Each UCV 1 book uses a series of approximately 100 **"supra-prototypical" cases as a way to condense testable facts and associations**. The clinical vignettes in this series are designed to incorporate as many testable facts as possible into a cohesive and memorable clinical picture. The vignettes represent composites drawn from general and specialty textbooks, reference books, thousands of USMLE style questions and the personal experience of the authors and reviewers.

Although each case tends to present all the signs, symptoms, and diagnostic findings for a particular illness, **patients generally will not present with such a "complete" picture either clinically or on a medical examination**. Cases are not meant to simulate a potential real patient or an exam vignette. All the **boldfaced "buzzwords" are for learning purposes** and are not necessarily expected to be found in any one patient with the disease.

Definitions of selected important terms are placed within the vignettes in (SMALL CAPS) in parentheses. Other parenthetical remarks often refer to the pathophysiology or mechanism of disease. The format should also help students learn to present cases succinctly during oral "bullet" presentations on clinical rotations. The cases are meant to serve as a condensed review, not as a primary reference. The information provided in this book has been prepared with a great deal of thought and careful research. This book should not, however, be considered as your sole source of information. Corrections, suggestions and submissions of new cases are encouraged and will be acknowledged and incorporated when appropriate in future editions.

ABBREVIATIONS

5-ASA	5-aminosalicylic acid
ABGs	arterial blood gases
ABVD	adriamycin/bleomycin/vincristine/dacarbazine
ACE	angiotensin-converting enzyme
ACTH	adrenocorticotropic hormone
ADH	antidiuretic hormone
AFP	alpha fetal protein
AI	aortic insufficiency
AIDS	acquired immunodeficiency syndrome
ALL	acute lymphocytic leukemia
ALT	alanine transaminase
AML	acute myelogenous leukemia
ANA	antinuclear antibody
ARDS	adult respiratory distress syndrome
ASD	atrial septal defect
ASO	anti-streptolysin O
AST	aspartate transaminase
AV	arteriovenous
BE	barium enema
BP	blood pressure
BUN	blood urea nitrogen
CAD	coronary artery disease
CALLA	common acute lymphoblastic leukemia antigen
CBC	complete blood count
CHF	congestive heart failure
CK	creatine kinase
CLL	chronic lymphocytic leukemia
CML	chronic myelogenous leukemia
CMV	cytomegalovirus
CNS	central nervous system
COPD	chronic obstructive pulmonary disease
CPK	creatine phosphokinase
CSF	cerebrospinal fluid
CT	computed tomography
CVA	cerebrovascular accident
CXR	chest x-ray
DIC	disseminated intravascular coagulation
DIP	distal interphalangeal
DKA	diabetic ketoacidosis
DM	diabetes mellitus
DTRs	deep tendon reflexes
DVT	deep venous thrombosis

EBV	Epstein–Barr virus
ECG	electrocardiography
Echo	echocardiography
EF	ejection fraction
EGD	esophagogastroduodenoscopy
EMG	electromyography
ERCP	endoscopic retrograde cholangiopancreatography
ESR	erythrocyte sedimentation rate
FEV	forced expiratory volume
FNA	fine needle aspiration
FTA-ABS	fluorescent treponemal antibody absorption
FVC	forced vital capacity
GFR	glomerular filtration rate
GH	growth hormone
GI	gastrointestinal
GM-CSF	granulocyte macrophage colony stimulating factor
GU	genitourinary
HAV	hepatitis A virus
hcG	human chorionic gonadotrophin
HEENT	head, eyes, ears, nose, and throat
HIV	human immunodeficiency virus
HLA	human leukocyte antigen
HPI	history of present illness
HR	heart rate
HRIG	human rabies immune globulin
HS	hereditary spherocytosis
ID/CC	identification and chief complaint
IDDM	insulin-dependent diabetes mellitus
Ig	immunoglobulin
IGF	insulin-like growth factor
IM	intramuscular
JVP	jugular venous pressure
KUB	kidneys/ureter/bladder
LDH	lactate dehydrogenase
LES	lower esophageal sphincter
LFTs	liver function tests
LP	lumbar puncture
LV	left ventricular
LVH	left ventricular hypertrophy
Lytes	electrolytes
MCHC	mean corpuscular hemoglobin concentration
MCV	mean corpuscular volume
MEN	multiple endocrine neoplasia

MGUS	monoclonal gammopathy of undetermined significance
MHC	major histocompatibility complex
MI	myocardial infarction
MOPP	mechlorethamine/vincristine (Oncovorin)/procarbazine/prednisone
MR	magnetic resonance (imaging)
NHL	non-Hodgkin's lymphoma
NIDDM	non-insulin-dependent diabetes mellitus
NPO	nil per os (nothing by mouth)
NSAID	nonsteroidal anti-inflammatory drug
PA	posteroanterior
PIP	proximal interphalangeal
PBS	peripheral blood smear
PE	physical exam
PFTs	pulmonary function tests
PMI	point of maximal intensity
PMN	polymorphonuclear leukocyte
PT	prothrombin time
PTCA	percutaneous transluminal angioplasty
PTH	parathyroid hormone
PTT	partial thromboplastin time
PUD	peptic ulcer disease
RBC	red blood cell
RPR	rapid plasma reagin
RR	respiratory rate
RS	Reed–Sternberg (cell)
RV	right ventricular
RVH	right ventricular hypertrophy
SBFT	small bowel follow-through
SIADH	syndrome of inappropriate secretion of ADH
SLE	systemic lupus erythematosus
STD	sexually transmitted disease
TFTs	thyroid function tests
tPA	tissue plasminogen activator
TSH	thyroid-stimulating hormone
TIBC	total iron-binding capacity
TIPS	transjugular intrahepatic portosystemic shunt
TPO	thyroid peroxidase
TSH	thyroid-stimulating hormone
TTP	thrombotic thrombocytopenic purpura
UA	urinalysis
UGI	upper GI
US	ultrasound

VDRL	Venereal Disease Research Laboratory
VS	vital signs
VT	ventricular tachycardia
WBC	white blood cell
WPW	Wolff–Parkinson–White (syndrome)
XR	x-ray

ID/CC	A 30-year-old man who is known to have **full-blown AIDS** presents with **tremor, ataxia, memory loss, and both visual and auditory hallucinations**.
HPI	He has no history of seizures, fever, neck stiffness, or vomiting.
PE	No focal neurologic signs; fundus normal; no meningeal signs.
Labs	LP: normal proteins in CSF; normal glucose. India ink staining negative (rule out cryptococcal meningitis); VDRL nonreactive (rule out neurosyphilis).
Imaging	MR, brain: bright spots (on T2 weighted); cortical atrophy and ventricular dilatation.
Gross Pathology	Diffuse leukoencephalopathy with enlargement of cortical sulci and ventricles.
Treatment	Antiretroviral therapy such as **zidovudine** may improve neuropsychiatric symptoms; no definitive treatment available.
Discussion	AIDS dementia complex is characterized by a **progressive dementia, psychomotor abnormalities, focal motor abnormalities, and behavioral changes**. Clinical manifestations of this disorder are found in at least two-thirds of patients with AIDS. However, neurologic manifestations in the HIV-infected individual may be associated with CNS disease caused by such organisms as *Cryptococcus neoformans, Toxoplasma gondii, Treponema pallidum,* and JC virus (progressive multifocal leukoencephalopathy) as well as with B-cell lymphoma.

AIDS DEMENTIA

ID/CC An 18-year-old man in the postdrome of a 12-day admission due to herpes simplex encephalitis reports anxiety caused by an **inability to recall events that occurred just before his hospitalization.**

HPI He also reports tingling of the buttocks since his illness.

Discussion Amnestic disorder often occurs as a result of pathologic processes (e.g., closed head trauma, penetrating wounds, surgical intervention, hypoxia, infarction of the posterior cerebral artery and its distributions, and encephalitis) that cause damage to specific diencephalic and mediotemporal lobe structures, such as the mammillary bodies, fornices, and hippocampus. **Herpes simplex infection is the most common cause of viral encephalitis in teenagers and young adults.** Amnesia may be transient (less than 1 month in duration) or chronic.

ID/CC   A 14-year-old male is brought by his neighbor to the ER after being found in a **confused, hostile state** with a cut over his right eye.

HPI   Further questioning of the neighbor reveals that the patient and his friend had been **inhaling turpentine** in the neighbor's garage. The boy was brought to the neighbor's attention after he exhibited strange behavior.

Treatment   **Haloperidol**, a neuroleptic, should be given as a sedative. Because the patient is under 18 years of age, child protective services should be contacted. The child's family should be informed about his actions and counseled.

3   **DELIRIUM—INHALANT ABUSE**

ID/CC	A **72-year-old** white woman hospitalized for 2 days with lobar pneumonia is restrained because of her **attempts to rise from bed** and pull out an IV line.
HPI	She appears **confused and anxious** and responds to questions with **rambling, incoherent speech**. Before her hospitalization, she had been living on her own. Her daughter denies any recent change in her mother's ability to take care of herself and **denies any use of drugs or alcohol** by her mother.
PE	VS: fever (39°C). PE: mini-mental status exams over past 2 days suggest **fluctuations in attention, orientation, and cognitive ability with generalized progressive degeneration**; consolidation in lower left lung with rales throughout.
Imaging	CT, head: normal.
Treatment	As many cues as possible should be supplied to allow patient to maintain a sense of time and place as well as a sense of security. If possible, a familiar family member or a 24-hour sitter should stay with patient at all times. A clock, calendar, or television may be used to orient patient to waking and sleeping hours. A neuroleptic agent (e.g., haloperidol) can be used if necessary to control agitation. Attempts should be made to eliminate underlying medical cause (e.g., infections or polypharmacy).
Discussion	Delirium is especially common in the elderly.

ID/CC	A 63-year-old male complains to his family physician of **progressive memory impairment**.
HPI	The patient **cannot remember his home address**. His wife reports that he was forced to stop working because he was making an increasing number of mistakes. She also reports a few brief episodes during which he has appeared dazed and uncommunicative.
PE	VS: BP normal. PE: no evidence of organic CNS pathology; **recent memory impairment on mental status exam** without impaired consciousness.
Imaging	CT, head: diffuse atrophy and prominent sulci.
Micro Pathology	**Neurofibrillary tangles** and **amyloid plaque** development are commonly seen in neurons of hippocampus.
Treatment	No specific cure; supportive management; caregiver counseling; tetrahydroaminoacridine (THAA), which was recently approved by the FDA, may have some benefit.
Discussion	Characterized by **degeneration of cholinergic neurons in the nucleus basalis**. The APP gene on chromosome 21 has been shown to be defective in a small subset of Alzheimer's patients. Alzheimer's disease is the most common cause of dementia in people over age 65.
Atlas Links	U C V 1 PG-BS-005, PM-BS-005A, PM-BS-005B

ID/CC	A 67-year-old woman is brought to the ER by her daughter because of a **sudden** diminishment in cognitive ability and left-sided gait disturbance.
HPI	Her daughter reports that the patient "was fine just this morning."
PE	VS: irregular pulse; **hypertension**. PE: mini-mental status exam score 22/30; speech slurred; neurologic examination reveals left leg paresthesia, weakness of flexor and extensor muscles, and diminished reflexes.
Labs	Normal motor conductance in muscles of left leg on EMG.
Imaging	MR: multiple small **cerebral infarctions**.
Treatment	Supportive treatment and rehabilitation.
Discussion	Patients with multi-infarct dementia exhibit **stepwise decline in mental function** (due to multiple small infarctions).

ID/CC   A 15-year-old white male presents with a 3-month history of **sudden, brief, irrepressible daytime sleep attacks, bilateral loss of muscle tone** (CATAPLEXY), and recurrent episodes of **REM sleep within minutes of falling asleep**.

HPI   He sometimes has **dreamlike auditory or visual hallucinations** while falling asleep (HYPNAGOGIC) and awakening (HYPNOPOMPIC). Occasionally he finds himself **paralyzed** for a few seconds **while awakening**. He denies any drug use and is not on any medications.

PE   Physical examination normal.

Labs   Sleep apnea or loud snoring may be present; EEG shows that patient's sleep cycle begins with REM sleep.

Treatment   **Methylphenidate**, a stimulant, may be used to prevent daytime sleep. **Imipramine** may be added if cataplexy is a significant component of the disorder. Benzodiazepines may be used to control insomnia, which can accompany presenting symptoms. Continuous positive airway pressure (CPAP) may be helpful in some cases if sleep apnea is involved.

Discussion   Narcolepsy affects roughly 1 in every 2000 people and is associated with a strong genetic component. The differential includes myxedema, hypercapnia, brain tumor, Kleine-Levin syndrome (hyperphagia, hypersomnia, and hypersexuality), and Pickwickian syndrome (obesity with respiratory insufficiency). The **patient progresses from an awake and alert state of consciousness directly into REM sleep**. Sleep attacks last for about 5 minutes.

ID/CC A **10-year-old** male **"spaces out"** during class and exhibits a slight quivering of his lips.

HPI These **brief seizures** happen several times a day, each lasting from a few seconds to a minute. The boy's teachers report that the child exhibits **no postictal confusion** but add that at times he **does not know that he has had a seizure**. He wears a helmet to prevent injury in the event of a seizure while walking.

Labs EEG: **3-Hz spikes and slow-wave activity**.

Imaging MR, brain: normal.

Treatment Pharmacologic therapy with **ethosuximide** and/or valproic acid.

Discussion Seizures tend to occur in childhood and often resolve with age. They should be differentiated from conversion disorders and dissociative disorders.

ID/CC A 25-year-old male is brought to the ER in a **drowsy state**; according to his wife, he was working in the house when he **suddenly lost consciousness** and fell to the ground.

HPI His wife reports that after he lost consciousness, his **respiration temporarily ceased**. This episode lasted for about 45 seconds and was **followed by jerking of all four limbs** for about 3 to 4 minutes. The patient was then unconscious for an additional 3 to 4 minutes. He has no history of fever, neck stiffness, or vomiting.

PE VS: normal. PE: large laceration on lip; fundus normal; no meningeal signs; no focal neurologic deficit; vitals maintained.

Labs Lytes: normal. Blood glucose normal. EEG: **normal background interrupted by generalized spike and slow-wave discharges** ranging from 3 to 5 Hz; can be elicited by hyperventilation, photic stimulation, and sleep.

Imaging CT, head: normal.

Treatment Anticonvulsant therapy with phenytoin or valproate.

Discussion A seizure is a paroxysmal, abnormal discharge of neurons of the cerebral cortex that alters neurologic function. Epilepsy is a heterogeneous condition characterized by recurrent, unprovoked seizures. More than 10% of the population of the United States will have a seizure at some time during their lives, and epilepsy will develop in 1% to 2% of the population.

ID/CC	A 40-year-old woman presents with a history of seizures characterized by an **aura of foul odor** at onset followed by **isolated jerking of the right thumb** and then the right hand, **spreading to the right arm** and then to the right side of the face without any loss of consciousness.
HPI	She states that she has **never lost consciousness** during any of her seizures.
PE	**No focal neurologic deficit** noted during interictal period.
Labs	EEG: regularly occurring spike discharges in left motor cortex during interictal period.
Treatment	**Carbamazepine** is drug of choice; newer agents such as gabapentin or lamotrigine may be useful.
Discussion	Simple-partial seizures **begin locally in the brain and spread outward to adjacent cortical structures**. They can be motor, sensory, autonomic, or psychic and may secondarily generalize.

SEIZURE, JACKSONIAN TYPE

ID/CC A 35-year-old woman presents with a 14-month history of episodes in which she loses contact with her surroundings.

HPI The patient's first episode was brought to her attention by a friend, who noticed that she **suddenly got a vague look in her eyes and started smacking her lips** and rubbing her right thumb against her left hand for 20 to 60 seconds. In recent months, the patient has also noticed a **foul odor and taste in her mouth**.

PE No focal neurologic signs.

Labs EEG: left-sided spikes; **sharp wave discharges over frontotemporal regions** both interictally and during seizure.

Imaging PET: temporal lobe hypometabolism interictally.

Treatment Carbamazepine is drug of choice; newer agents such as gabapentin or lamotrigine may be useful.

Discussion Temporal lobe epilepsy can present with a **wide range of abnormal behaviors**, including labile affect, auditory hallucinations, and even paranoid ideation.

ID/CC A 33-year-old male arrives in the ER in **continuous seizure**.

HPI Upon regaining consciousness after a period of **postictal confusion**, he reports that he was **previously diagnosed with epilepsy** and recently **stopped taking his medication**.

PE Examination to rule out heart disease, meningitis, and increased intracranial pressure produces no findings; no papilledema; no nuchal rigidity on passive neck flexion.

Labs EEG: **typical epileptic spikes**. ECG: regular sinus rhythm. LP: normal opening pressure; slightly elevated protein.

Imaging CT, head: no intracranial bleeding or mass lesions.

Treatment Status epilepticus is a **medical emergency**; IV diazepam or lorazepam should be administered immediately. Prolonged status epilepticus can result in permanent brain damage. After the acute event has resolved, preventive pharmacologic therapy should be started. Carbamazepine, phenytoin, primidone, and phenobarbital have all been used with some success.

Discussion The differential diagnosis includes meningitis, brain abscess, stroke, head trauma, metabolic disturbances (e.g., hyponatremia), drug reaction, alcohol/anticonvulsant drug withdrawal, vitamin B_6 deficiency, and panic attack.

ID/CC A 17-year-old male is brought to the ER by the police because of cold exposure; he had casually left his parents' home after **destroying furniture** and appliances in their living room **following an argument** they had had about his curfew.

HPI Interview of his parents reveals that the young man is a **promising student** but has had disciplinary problems at school and at home. This episode marked **the most exaggerated and aggressive of his many outbursts**, although it is characterized by lack of emotion on his part.

PE VS: tachycardia; skin cold and clammy (due to peripheral vasoconstriction).

Discussion Acting out is an action-level **ego defense mechanism** in which the individual **deals with emotional conflict or internal or external stressors through actions rather than reflections or feelings**. Acting out should be differentiated from other inappropriate behavior on the basis of evidence relating behavior to emotional conflict.

ID/CC   A 35-year-old male is diagnosed with ischemic heart disease following an evaluation for an episode of anginal chest pain; on the following day he is **found doing push-ups prior to a medical consultation**.

HPI   On further interview, he states that there is **"nothing wrong" with him** and that "it's all just an overreaction."

Discussion   The defense mechanism employed here is denial. The patient finds it difficult to believe he is ill and uses **denial to cope** with the difficult news of his illness.

ID/CC A 34-year-old woman presenting for her annual gynecologic exam erupts into tears upon hearing that her Pap smear showed atypical cells, announcing between sobs that "things like this always happen" to her.

HPI She rejects attempts to comfort her, stating that "that's the way things are; stupid things happen to useless people." She continues by calling herself a whore and states that the finding is an appropriate punishment for the sexual promiscuity of her youth.

Discussion Devaluation is an image-distorting ego defense mechanism in which an **individual deals with emotional conflict or internal or external stressors by attributing exaggerated negative qualities to self**.

ID/CC A physician seeing her first patient of the day is **uncharacteristically forceful** in advising that patient to lose weight.

HPI She had an **argument with her son** the previous night, during which he again refused to take what she considered to be sound advice.

Discussion The defense mechanism being used by the physician is displacement. Displacement involves the **transfer of emotions** from an **unacceptable to an acceptable person or object** and has been associated with the development of phobias in psychodynamic theory.

DISPLACEMENT

ID/CC A 27-year-old male professional presents to the internist for a work physical; the visit proceeds normally until the subject of his sexual history arises, at which time the patient becomes **overtly shy**, no longer looks directly at the examiner, and begins to **giggle**.

HPI Further inquiry about past sexual activity only enhances his shy behavior. **Normal mature behavior returns** with continuation of the remaining history.

PE Physical exam normal; patient again demonstrates shy and embarrassed behavior during the urogenital exam.

Discussion Fixation is an ego defense mechanism marked by a partial or localized **paralysis at a more childish level of development**.

ID/CC	A 37-year-old woman presents with lower abdominal pain, lethargy, and pain on defecation.
HPI	Questioning reveals that the patient's **symptoms began soon after her spouse's death** from colon cancer.
PE	Abdomen tender to palpation.
Labs	Stool guaiac negative.
Imaging	Colonoscopy reveals no abnormalities.
Treatment	Psychotherapy may be beneficial.
Discussion	Identification is an **ego defense mechanism** in which a person's **behavior is unconsciously patterned after someone else**; it is often associated with **child abuse or loss**.

ID/CC A 24-year-old medical student recounts his experience in gross anatomy to his family over the Thanksgiving holiday.

HPI His **emotionless and scientific narrative** is interrupted by his sister's surprise that he has **not harbored any of the concern and guilt** that he had expected to encounter in the process of dissection.

Discussion Isolation of affect is an **inhibitory ego defense mechanism** characterized by a **separation of feelings from ideas and events**.

ID/CC	A 28-year-old man presents for an annual physical; after testing positive for gonorrhea, he reveals that he has been cheating on his wife, stating that **she cares more about her career than she cares about him**.
HPI	He loves his wife and feels compatible with her, but while she was struggling to earn a promotion, he engaged in numerous affairs.
Treatment	Psychotherapy can help by bringing true issues out so that they can be discussed.
Discussion	Rationalization is a **subconscious process** in which a person **relieves some of his or her anxieties** about doing something socially unacceptable **by providing a logical reason for doing it**.

ID/CC A 15-year-old boy being seen for a sports physical reveals his disgust at his best friend's confession that he might be gay, stating that he "can't stand being near that faggot" and that "all homosexuals should go to hell."

HPI He and the young man have been best friends for years; he admits that he has never been closer to anyone else. He appears shaken by the process of recounting his experience.

Discussion Reaction formation is an **inhibitory ego defense mechanism** marked by the **replacement of a personally unacceptable idea or feeling by an emphasis on its opposite**. In this case, the patient has structured a strong homophobia to deny any possibility of attraction to his male friend.

ID/CC   A 24-year-old woman with a history of systemic lupus erythema-tosus (SLE) **begins bedwetting** and **throwing tantrums** at her biweekly appointments for dialysis.

HPI   Since being diagnosed with SLE, she has had to leave graduate school and **move in with her parents**. She has found dialysis to be a painful and very trying experience and often **sucks her thumb** to ease her anxiety.

Discussion   Regression is characterized by **childlike behavior under stress**, such as physical illness or hospitalization.

ID/CC	A witness of an appalling crime visits his physician because he **cannot recall** any details about the assailant.
HPI	Despite the patient's repeated efforts, he cannot elicit this memory.
Treatment	Hypnosis has proven useful in some cases.
Discussion	**Repression is the involuntary exclusion of painful memories** or impulses from awareness. **Suppression is the exclusion of painful memories or impulses resulting from conscious effort** (e.g., to stop thinking about an upsetting event without actually forgetting that event).

DEFENSE MECHANISM

REPRESSION

ID/CC   A patient who has been hospitalized for coronary bypass surgery describes the house staff as either **angelic or demonic**.

HPI   Further questioning reveals that this **dichotomy** also encompasses the patient's understanding of his **relationship to his family and to people at work**.

Discussion   Splitting involves a **compartmentalization of opposite affect states to deal with emotional conflict or internal or external stressors**. Because ambivalent affects cannot be experienced simultaneously, the patient's emotional awareness rests on an exclusion of balanced views and expectations of self and others. **Often seen in patients with personality disorders, especially borderline personality**.

ID/CC   A 27-year-old man tells his physician of his decision to go into civic law upon his graduation from law school this summer.

HPI   He plans to pursue a career in criminal prosecution law despite his father's desire that he enter a more lucrative field. He repeatedly mentions that his brother was killed by a drunk driver who received a minimal sentence.

Discussion   In sublimation, an **unacceptable instinctual impulse is channeled into a socially acceptable action**. Here, the unacceptable desire for vengeance through vigilantism was channeled into a desire to become a criminal prosecutor. Considered a "mature" defense mechanism.

SUBLIMATION

ID/CC A 28-year-old woman presents with a 3-month history of **anxiety and depression following her breakup with her fiancé** of 3 years.

HPI She has been **overwhelmed by feelings of sadness, tearfulness, and depression** and is concerned that she will never be in a relationship again or fulfill her dream of having a family. Since her breakup with her fiancé, she has **lost touch with friends and family**, and her **performance at work has steadily declined**.

PE Physical exam reveals a cachectic and poorly groomed woman.

Discussion Adjustment disorder (AD) is characterized by the **development of clinically significant emotional or behavioral symptoms in response to an identifiable psychosocial stressor or stressors**. The symptoms must develop within 3 months after the onset of the stressor. ADs are coded according to the subtype that best characterizes the predominant symptoms. In this case, the patient would be diagnosed as adjustment disorder with mixed anxiety and depressed mood.

ID/CC A female patient complains of **uncontrollable anxiety of more than 6 months' duration** together with daily symptoms that she attributes to a heart condition.

HPI The symptoms interfere with her social and professional life because she never knows when the anxiety will begin. She is **irritable, fatigues easily, has poor concentration**, and has **difficulty falling asleep**. She reports that during the exacerbations, her heart beats quickly, she sweats, and she occasionally has diarrhea. The patient has no specific phobias.

Labs Normal cardiac enzymes. ECG: regular sinus rhythm. Normal TSH level.

Treatment Buspirone; some patients may benefit from short-term low-dose benzodiazepines; antidepressants may also confer benefit, particularly selective serotonin reuptake inhibitors (SSRIs). Patients should be counseled to maintain a productive lifestyle. Acute anxiety can be managed with biofeedback and meditation. Heart palpitations may be controlled with beta-blockers.

Discussion In roughly half of all patients, the disorder resolves with time. Before diagnosing generalized anxiety disorder, **rule out thyroid disorders and pheochromocytoma**.

GENERALIZED ANXIETY DISORDER

ID/CC	A 21-year-old female student having a routine physical exam appears distracted and focused on the office ceiling; when confronted by the physician, she is embarrassed but admits that she is **counting the number of tiles on the ceiling**.
HPI	For the past 5 months, she has experienced an **irresistible urge to count objects** on a daily basis. She estimates that she spends 1 to 2 hours counting tiles each morning, often **missing her classes or meetings** as a result. The patient adds that she is **distressed by the unreasonable amount of time** she spends on such activities but feels that she can't stop. She denies any substance abuse or use of medications.
Labs	Lab work normal.
Treatment	**Exposure therapy** and other types of **behavioral therapy** have been proven useful. Obsessive-compulsive disorder (OCD) may involve dysfunction of cortical **serotonin** systems. **Clomipramine**, a tricyclic antidepressant, has been shown to have an effect on OCD symptoms. **Selective serotonin reuptake inhibitors (SSRIs)** are also useful.
Discussion	The prevalence of obsessive-compulsive disorder is estimated to be 1%. Onset occurs most often in adolescence or early adulthood. This disorder can manifest itself in the form of **compulsive habits** or **persistent thoughts or images** that are perceived as **intrusive** (obsessions) and that cause the patient significant distress.

OBSESSIVE-COMPULSIVE DISORDER

ID/CC A 57-year-old man is brought to the ER following an episode of **chest pain, dizziness, diaphoresis, and shortness of breath** which ended in syncope.

HPI He is somewhat confused by his arrival at the hospital. Workup reveals **no signs of MI**. Further questioning reveals that the patient has had **numerous such episodes** in the past, each preceded by **thoughts of speaking before the executive board** of his company.

Labs ECG: no ST depression or elevation; no other evidence of myocardial damage.

Treatment Benzodiazepines to alleviate acute symptoms. Behavioral therapy (systematic desensitization and cognitive therapy) has shown success in enabling the individual to counteract anxiety brought about by panic triggers.

Discussion Panic disorder is **characterized by discrete periods of intense fear or discomfort** peaking in 10 minutes with four of the following: (1) palpitations and racing heart; (2) sweating; (3) trembling; (4) shortness of breath; (5) choking feeling; (6) chest pain; (7) nausea/abdominal distress; (8) dizziness, faintness, and lightheadedness; (9) derealization; (10) fear of losing control; (11) fear of dying; (12) paresthesias; and (13) chills or hot flashes. Panic disorder must be diagnosed in a certain context, e.g., panic disorder with agoraphobia. In this case, the patient's panic attack was elicited by his fear of public speaking.

PANIC DISORDER

ID/CC   A war veteran complains of **intense and vivid flashbacks** with associated **anxiety and hyperarousal**.

HPI   The patient has **witnessed and experienced traumatic events** but **cannot recall** certain details of these events, and he **becomes anxious** both when questioned about the events and **when he encounters cues that remind him of them**. He also reports **difficulty falling asleep, hypervigilance, emotional outbursts, difficulty concentrating, and recurrent nightmares** that have begun to **interfere with his life**.

PE   Patient appears anxious.

Treatment   Counseling should begin as soon after the traumatic event as possible. Some patients may benefit from benzodiazepines (for anxiety) and antidepressants.

Discussion   Seventy-five percent of patients drop out of counseling programs because remembering the traumatic event is too anxiety-provoking. PTSD may be classified as **acute (duration of 3 months or less)** or **chronic (duration of more than 3 months)**.

ID/CC A 36-year-old woman tells her physician that **she turned down a promotion at work** because her new duties would have included **speaking in front of the company's executive board**.

HPI She is upset about her decision but maintains that she **"just couldn't get up in front of them."**

Treatment **Cognitive behavioral psychotherapy** is the most effective treatment; MAO inhibitors and selective serotonin reuptake inhibitors (SSRIs) may be helpful for generalized social phobia. Beta-blockers or benzodiazepines may alleviate anxiety on an as-needed basis in specific social phobias (e.g., test-taking or performance anxiety).

Discussion Exposure to the feared situation almost invariably causes anxiety in patients with social phobia. The individual recognizes that the fear is an unreasonable one. Frequent comorbidity with substance abuse and depression.

SOCIAL PHOBIA

ID/CC   An 8-year-old male is brought to the family physician by his mother because he makes careless mistakes, **cannot maintain his concentration or listen to commands**, and is forgetful, hyperactive, and noisy.

HPI   He has been like this for **at least 6 months**. He also shows **poor impulse control**. His performance in school has suffered, and he has few friends. There is no history of psychosis.

PE   Patient appears restless and **fidgets continuously**; physical and mental development normal for age.

Treatment   **Treatment of choice** is a **stimulant**, most commonly methylphenidate (Ritalin), and supportive family therapy.

Discussion   There are three types of ADHD: **attention-deficit predominant type**, formerly known as attention deficit disorder (ADD); **hyperactivity predominant type**; and **combined type**. Children with ADHD are often placed in classes for those with learning disabilities because they are unable to concentrate.

ID/CC	A 4-year-old boy presents with **severe language delay** together with an **inability to interact with other children or adults**; his parents say that he spends a great deal of time **spinning around in circles**.
HPI	His parents state that they noticed nothing unusual in infancy except the child's **indifference to being cuddled**.
PE	Physical development normal; intelligence subnormal; child is **not interactive** and exhibits **repetitive behavior**.
Labs	Serum serotonin level elevated; other tests normal.
Treatment	Aim therapy at increasing social and communication skills and at improving self-care ability. Group therapy with autistic or normal peers may yield improved social function.
Discussion	Autistic disorder is a **pervasive developmental disorder** that begins before three years of age and is found in 0.05% of all children. Of these, only 2% can live independently; most remain severely impaired throughout their lives. Children with pure mental retardation can be distinguished from those with infantile autism in that they do not exhibit bizarre behavior or deficits in social relations.

AUTISM

ID/CC	A 10-month-old female is brought to the doctor by her mother, who feels that the baby is retarded, cannot see properly, and falls repeatedly; the child has **bruises in different stages of healing** (suggestive of child abuse).
PE	No lacerations or fractures noted; normal physical development for 10 months of age; **bilateral retinal hemorrhages** seen; skin, sclera, joints normal.
Labs	Coagulation profile normal.
Imaging	XR: no old or new fractures seen.
Treatment	**Health care workers are required by law to report any suspicion of child abuse or neglect to state protection agencies**; victims are immediately removed from homes and placed in protective custody of a hospital or state facility.
Discussion	Vigorous shaking can produce **vitreous and retinal hemorrhages** that may be the only verifiable signs of child abuse.
Atlas Link	ⓊⒸⓋ2 PED-053

ID/CC	A 10-year-old schoolboy is brought in for a consultation because he **fails to follow school rules** and shows **no concern for the feelings of others**.
HPI	He has been known to trick his fellow students into giving him their lunch money. His teacher feels that he suffers from a behavioral disorder and needs psychiatric treatment.
PE	Physical exam normal; physical and mental development normal for age.
Labs	Routine tests within normal range.
Treatment	Behavioral therapy.
Discussion	Conduct disorder involves **failure to follow social norms** and **corresponds to an increased risk of criminal behavior in adults**. Associated with antisocial personality disorder in adulthood.

ID/CC A **6-year-old boy** is brought by his mother to the family physician because of a **7-month history of episodic bedwetting**.

HPI The child is **ashamed** to talk about his experience. His mother reports that his **performance in school has markedly decreased** in the past months. He has no history of seizures or spina bifida.

Labs Fasting blood glucose level normal (rule out juvenile diabetes).

Treatment Therapy should be directed toward both the problem itself and its psychological consequences.

Discussion Enuresis is defined as **urinary incontinence that is not due to a medical condition**. It may be voluntary or involuntary and can occur during the day or, more commonly, at night. Differential diagnosis should include neurogenic bladder, medical conditions that cause polyuria or urgency (e.g., juvenile diabetes, spina bifida, seizure disorder), and acute UTI. **Most children with the disorder become continent by adolescence**.

ID/CC	A 4-year-old girl is brought to the physician by her drug-abusing mother for an evaluation of **developmental delay**, repetitive play, and **underdeveloped language skills**.
HPI	Although the patient's mother abstained from drug and alcohol use during pregnancy, her mother and father frequently became drunk and fought with each other after the child was born. Often the patient was caught in the middle. The mother reports that the patient frequently comes to her in the middle of the night complaining **of bad dreams**. The mother has also noted **repetitive destructive behavior**. The patient often locks her doll in the closet and, upon hearing sirens, runs around tearfully and screams. She is **hypervigilant** with strangers and is **easily startled**.
Treatment	The most important aspect of treatment is ensuring safe home environment. Psychotherapy and tutoring are also beneficial.
Discussion	Adults with PTSD can often describe clear flashbacks. Children, however, generally lack the ability to understand and communicate their experiences as clearly, and diagnosis must therefore be based on history and play observation. **Disorganized or agitated behavior, repetitive play**, or **frightening dreams** may be observed.

POST-TRAUMATIC STRESS DISORDER (CHILD)

ID/CC	A 5-year-old child develops **abdominal pain every Monday morning**.
HPI	The child does not report any abnormality in his stools, and his parents have not noted any irregularity in his eating habits.
Labs	Routine hemogram and stool exam fail to detect any abnormality.
Treatment	Mild school avoidance should be managed with encouragement and by sending the child to school unless symptoms of illness are found. In more severe cases, a psychiatric referral should be made.
Discussion	A child with separation anxiety may develop **functional symptoms** on days when he has to go to school; he feigns illness because it will keep him at home. Genetic factors, learning disabilities, mental retardation, and developmental immaturity may contribute to separation anxiety.

ID/CC	A 47-year-old patient is referred by her family physician to a psychiatrist because her husband is concerned about a series of recent episodes in which the patient has **awoken screaming or crying** in the middle of the night.
HPI	Her husband's attempts to awaken and comfort her are fruitless, and she gradually returns to peaceful sleep and **remembers nothing the next morning**. The episodes have been occurring every 3 to 4 days; however, they occurred every night while the patient's daughter was hospitalized for pneumonia.
Treatment	Stress reduction measures and psychiatric evaluation.
Discussion	Most patients do not awaken fully and have **amnesia for the episode in the morning**. Patients who do not experience amnesia for sleep terrors report fragmented fearful images rather than a storylike sequence (observed in nightmares). Sleep terrors **occur in delta sleep**, and patients exhibit intense fear and **autonomic arousal. Episode frequency increases with stress.**

SLEEP TERRORS

ID/CC An 8-year-old **male** is brought to his pediatrician with complaints of **repeated eye blinking, head jerking, and shoulder shrugging** of 2 years' duration.

HPI The patient has never had a tic-free period for more than 1 month. Recently, he has started making **involuntary sounds** that begin as slight grunts but progress to **loud barks and obscenities**.

PE Involuntary tics.

Treatment **Haloperidol** is effective in controlling tics. Psychotherapy may relieve stressful situations that may serve as precipitating factors.

Discussion **Dysfunctional regulation of dopamine** is most commonly involved in Gilles de la Tourette syndrome. It affects males three times more often than females; onset is most common before age 21.

TIC DISORDERS—TOURETTE'S

ID/CC	A **17-year-old woman** presents with **amnesia** over a 3-hour period **following the death of a close friend**.
HPI	She reports no memory loss other than that concerning the period mentioned. She remembers in detail the last conversation she had with her friend but is **distressed** that she is unable to recall when her mother informed her of her friend's death. She **denies any substance abuse** or **recent physical trauma**.
Treatment	Hospitalization may be helpful to remove threatening stimulus; psychotherapy to examine loss of memory. Psychotherapy is often very successful.
Discussion	Dissociative amnesia is most common in adolescent and young adult females and is rare in the elderly. **Amnesia is localized and often follows a psychologically traumatic event**.

DISSOCIATIVE AMNESIA

ID/CC   A 24-year-old man presents with a history of **repeated episodes of anxiety-provoking detachment** during which he feels as if he is an external observer of his actions and thoughts.

HPI   These episodes have occurred intermittently over the past 14 months. He also reports having felt **depressed** for long periods of time throughout the past year.

Treatment   Pharmacologic interventions may be used for accompanying symptoms of anxiety, depression, or obsessions. Psychotherapy may be of value.

Discussion   Depersonalization can occur in a number of disorders, including post-traumatic stress disorder (PTSD), substance abuse, and seizure disorders. Dissociative disorder is diagnosed with **recurrent episodes in the absence of these other disorders**.

ID/CC	A 50-year-old woman who has lived in California all her life **discovers that she is in Texas** and **does not know how she got there**.
HPI	Her husband died in an automobile accident 2 weeks ago.
Treatment	Supportive psychotherapy.
Discussion	Dissociative fugue and dissociative amnesia both involve **failure to remember important information about oneself**. Dissociative fugue is further characterized by sudden, unexpected travel away from home with confusion about personal identity or even assumption of a new identity.

DISSOCIATIVE FUGUE

ID/CC   A 22-year-old woman presents to the emergency room in acute distress with a **2-hour history of amnesia** followed by what she describes as **"voices in her head"** telling her to kill herself.

HPI   She reports that these **amnesic episodes** have occurred before. She has tried to kill herself on two previous occasions, each time persuaded by the same voice that prompted her visit to the ER. She **denies any substance abuse** but has a **history of severe physical and emotional abuse as a child.**

PE   Sodium amylbarbital interview reveals second personality characterized by anger and disdain for patient's presenting personality; further questioning reveals that this personality has taken an active role in each of patient's suicide attempts.

Labs   **Shifts in personality correspond to changes in galvanic skin conductance, heart rate, muscle tone, visual acuity, and EEG wave patterns.**

Treatment   Psychotherapy and hypnotherapy should accompany medical therapy of associated disorders such as severe depression (selective serotonin reuptake inhibitors, tricyclics), psychoses (neuroleptics), and anxiety (benzodiazepines).

Discussion   Dissociative identity disorder was formerly referred to as **multiple personality disorder.**

DISSOCIATIVE IDENTITY DISORDER

ID/CC   A **14-year-old female** is brought to the physician by her mother because her **body weight is less than 85% of that expected** and she has **missed her last three periods** (AMENORRHEA).

HPI   The patient reports that she is fat and strongly fears gaining weight. She also reports intense hunger but prefers not to eat. She admits to abusing laxatives.

PE   Patient severely underweight.

Labs   Pregnancy test negative.

Treatment   Individual and family therapy along with antidepressant medication; in severe cases, hospitalization may be required.

Discussion   There are two major types of eating disorders: anorexia nervosa and bulimia. The current case describes anorexia nervosa. Females are 10 times more likely to be affected than males, and there is a higher incidence among those of upper to middle socioeconomic status. Anorexia nervosa has a 5% to 10% mortality rate.

ANOREXIA NERVOSA

ID/CC   A **20-year-old female college student** reveals a secret problem to her family physician.

HPI   She has always been preoccupied by her body. **Several times a week**, she suffers **uncontrollable eating binges**. She almost always follows these binges with a visit to the bathroom, where she discreetly **makes herself vomit**. Following each such episode, **she feels depressed**.

Treatment   Pharmacologic approach uses antidepressants; psychological approach uses psychotherapy, cognitive behavioral therapy.

Discussion   Bulimia nervosa is characterized by **binge eating followed by purging**, which is accomplished by self-induced vomiting, laxative use, or use of diuretics. The prevalence of this condition in the United States is approximately 1.5% among young women but is rarely seen in men. The typical patient is usually somewhat underweight and binges and purges several times a week. Dietary intake may be very restricted, with nonpurged caloric intake averaging 1,000 kcal/day. Depression is often comorbid.

ID/CC A 37-year-old man presents for a work physical **to document loss of vision** that arose after **exposure to a volatile toxin at the work site**.

HPI There is no significant medical history. He reports total intractable blindness since the accident at work and is **seeking disability payments** from the company he works for.

PE VS: normal. PE: visual field testing demonstrates apparent total visual loss. Pupils equal, round, and reactive to light and accommodation; patient's eyes move rapidly back and forth when asked to fixate on numbers of a tape measure while the tape is being rapidly pulled out (OPTOKINETIC NYSTAGMUS; verifies that patient is feigning blindness).

Discussion Malingering is defined as **feigning illness or disability to escape work, elicit sympathy, or gain compensation**.

MALINGERING

ID/CC A 37-year-old female with a history of insulin-dependent diabetes mellitus (IDDM) is admitted to the hospital for severe diabetic ketoacidosis (DKA).

HPI The patient is educated, articulate, and assertive and seems to be **extremely knowledgeable about her disease**. She claims that she controls her diabetes rigorously. After some phone inquiries, it is discovered that she has been admitted for hypoglycemia or DKA **at various local hospitals 23 times over the past 18 months**. When confronted with this finding, the patient becomes **angry and defensive** and leaves the hospital.

Labs Hyperglycemia (614 upon admission); HbA-1C 8% (elevation demonstrates poor long-term control of blood glucose).

Treatment It is important to **build rapport** when possible. The primary physician may want to interact with the patient in a **nonconfrontational** manner. Psychotherapy (with an emphasis on understanding etiology) may help, but the **prognosis is poor**.

Discussion Also known as **factitious disorder**, Munchausen's syndrome stems from a **conscious production of signs and symptoms of disease**. In this case, the patient's noncompliance was intentional. The aim of such patients is to **assume the sick role** when there is **no apparent benefit** to doing so.

MUNCHAUSEN'S SYNDROME

ID/CC A 10-year-old boy is brought to his family physician by his parents, who are concerned about his "feminine tendencies"; the boy's parents state that he continually **asks for clothes** and toys that are **designed for girls**, has **only female friends**, and on several occasions has been found **wearing his older sister's clothes**.

HPI The boy's parents claim that their son has always seemed to identify with the female gender. As a toddler, he protested at the prospect of being dressed in a suit and always sat while urinating. **The boy claims that he wants to be a girl** and adds that his favorite pastimes are games such as "house," in which he likes to **play "the wife."** His parents had hoped that he would grow out of this "phase" and are becoming increasingly concerned.

PE Physical exam unremarkable; normal male genitalia.

Treatment Adult patients may elect to undergo pharmacologic (e.g., estrogen) therapy or sex-reassignment surgery.

Discussion Gender identity disorder can be defined as a **persistent and powerful identification with the opposite gender**. It cannot stem from perceived social advantages associated with the other gender. Cross-gender behaviors tend not to continue into late adolescence. About three-fourths of such people subsequently report a bisexual or homosexual orientation. When gender identity continues into or begins in adulthood, it usually assumes a chronic course.

ID/CC A 40-year-old white female comes to the emergency room claiming that she is Jesus Christ.

HPI She is now medically stable and admits that she is not Jesus as "the voices" had told her. Over the past week, she has **slept fewer than 3 hours per night**. She initially excelled at work but recently became irritable and unable to concentrate. She then experienced **auditory command hallucinations** which told her that she had special powers. She recalls a similar episode several years ago and reports that occasionally she has felt depressed. She denies any drug use.

PE **Concentration impaired**; patient has flight of ideas; **speech rapid**; dressed in brightly colored clothes.

Labs TSH normal.

Treatment **Lithium** has been the traditional treatment of choice. Depakote and Tegretol are also effective treatments. Benzodiazepines and typical antipsychotic drugs may be useful short-term adjuncts.

Discussion More than 90% of bipolar disorder patients have a depressive episode. Manic episodes progress over days, and 20% of patients will have psychotic symptoms **(hallucinations and delusions)**. Women are four times more likely than men to be rapid cyclers (i.e., to have four or more manic and depressive cycles per year).

BIPOLAR I DISORDER, MANIC TYPE

ID/CC   A 28-year-old male writer being seen for a routine annual physical reports recent **irritability and insomnia**.

HPI   He states that he has been extremely productive lately and that his work has demonstrated the value of his enhanced alertness. Upon further questioning, he reveals that he experiences these **hyperenergetic states episodically**; they are often **followed by periods of malaise, apathy, loss of appetite, decreased ability to concentrate, and hypersomnia** (MAJOR DEPRESSIVE EPISODE). He has considered these fluctuations to be a normal consequence of his work.

PE   Physical exam reveals a hyperalert but otherwise normal-appearing man.

Discussion   Bipolar II disorder should be considered in any case in which **hypomanic disorder is accompanied by prodrome or postdrome depression** that meets the criteria for major depressive disorder. Hypomanic disorder is similar to a manic episode except that mood disturbances are not severe enough to cause marked impairment in social or occupational functioning.

BIPOLAR II DISORDER

ID/CC A 16-year-old girl is brought by her mother to her family physician because of **mood fluctuations and poor performance** in school for the past year.

HPI She reports week-long **episodes of tiredness and generalized unhappiness over several years** (DYSTHYMIA) followed by **short periods of high energy and euphoria**. Her older brother is receiving treatment for depression.

Discussion Cyclothymic disorder entails a **2-year history (1 year** in children and adolescents) of numerous periods of **hypomanic symptoms** preceded or followed by **periods marked by depressive symptoms** that do not meet the criteria for a major depressive episode. There is a 15% to 50% risk that the person will subsequently develop bipolar I or II disorder.

CYCLOTHYMIC DISORDER

ID/CC	An 80-year-old female who was recently diagnosed with breast cancer complains of **significant weight loss** and **forgetfulness** as well as multiple vague somatic complaints.
HPI	She was scheduled for a mastectomy, and she had been undergoing presurgical evaluation. Her best friend died a few days ago.
PE	Old, frail woman with hard lump in left breast; lymphadenopathy; no meningeal or focal neurologic signs; higher mental functions normal; no organomegaly found on abdominal exam; **admits to being depressed but denies any suicidal ideation**.
Treatment	Antidepressant medication, psychiatric consultation. Watch for side effects of antidepressants in the elderly (orthostatic hypotension with tricyclic antidepressants).
Discussion	The patient's recent and significant weight loss and her forgetfulness suggest that she is suffering from a major depressive episode. **Depression in the elderly often resembles pseudodementia** and can be treated effectively with antidepressant medication or electroconvulsive therapy.

DEPRESSION—ELDERLY

ID/CC   A 42-year-old woman is brought by the police to the ER following a failed suicide attempt.

HPI   The patient reports that she has felt **progressively sad** (DYSPHORIC) and **lacking in energy** over the past few months and has had **difficulty sleeping** over the same time period. She has **considered killing herself** numerous times but has only recently conceived of a plan by which to do so. She was recently fired because of her lethargy at work and has **lost interest in her long-time hobby** of reading. She feels **helpless** and **hopeless** about the state of her life and sees no solution other than to end it.

PE   Depressed mood; restricted affect; suicidal ideation.

Treatment   Assessment of suicide risk should be conducted before the patient is allowed to return home. Psychotherapy should accompany pharmacologic approaches to treatment of depression. Selective serotonin reuptake inhibitors (SSRIs) are considered first-line agents. Tricyclic agents and MAO inhibitors are considered second-line agents. Electroconvulsive therapy (ECT) is a consideration in recalcitrant and severe depression or if psychotic symptoms are present.

Discussion   Suicide attempt rates in major depression have been found to be between 15% and 30%. Providers should be aware that asking questions about suicide ideation does not increase the chance that suicide will occur.

ID/CC	A 50-year-old **female** attorney with a promising practice, two daughters, and a stable marriage is brought to her family physician for evaluation because her husband notes that she has "not been functioning properly" for the past 2 months.
HPI	She has called her office frequently to tell her colleagues that she is ill, whereas in fact she was **unable to get out of bed in the morning**. She has **ceased to take pride in her appearance**, has **lost her appetite for food and her interest in sex**, and has been **oversleeping** every day. She recently told her husband that she was **unsure whether she wanted to go on living**. She has no history of alcohol or other substance abuse.
PE	PE normal; **suicidal thoughts without plan** on mental status exam.
Labs	**Thyroid function tests normal**.
Treatment	Hospitalization and supervised antidepressant therapy.
Discussion	Major depressive episodes are two to three times more common in women than in men. In suicidal patients, consider an antidepressant that is safe in the event of overdose, such as selective serotonin reuptake inhibitors (SSRIs).

DEPRESSIVE EPISODE—MAJOR

ID/CC	A 38-year-old man reveals a three-year history of **depressed mood** during a routine physical exam; he states that he is **always tired and "feeling blue."**
HPI	The patient reports that he is doing fine at work but does not hope for advancement because "I'm just not good enough." He also states, **"I don't remember ever really being happy."** The patient reports **difficulty making decisions**. Upon questioning, he denies any suicidal ideation or substance abuse.
Labs	Normal T_3, T_4, and TSH (rule out hypothyroidism).
Treatment	Some patients respond to antidepressants. Treatment should focus on insight-oriented psychotherapy and behavioral therapy.
Discussion	Patients with dysthymic disorder exhibit **chronic (2+ years) depressed mood without clear onset**. The mood is persistent (only brief periods of normal mood) and often associated with **low self-esteem, hopelessness, pessimism, and low energy**.

DYSTHYMIC DISORDER

ID/CC A 30-year-old male is brought to the physician complaining that he wants to kill his fiancee's murderer and the emergency room doctors who couldn't save her.

HPI His fiancee was assaulted and died 2 days ago. During the interview, he repeatedly changes topics and talks about his fiancee's death. He frequently **alternates between apathy and anger** and **complains of vague GI discomfort** and **shortness of breath**. He also complains of **poor sleep**. He has no history of prolonged hysteria or inappropriate euphoria.

PE Patient is **restless and preoccupied** and **occasionally cries during examination; paresthesias** found that cannot be explained anatomically (SOMATIZATION DISORDER).

Treatment Medication to attenuate the normal grief process is not recommended. Small doses of **benzodiazepines for sleep** may be helpful in the short run. Patient should be allowed to grieve at his own pace. If patient is willing, he should be referred to a support group.

Discussion One-fourth of patients may experience symptoms of major depression during the first year of grief. One-tenth will have delusions or hallucinations. Some will develop somatization disorders, and others may abuse drugs or alcohol.

ID/CC	A 55-year-old male artist complains of suffering "terrible pangs of grief" since his wife died in an auto collision 5 months ago; he claims that he is **unable to think of anything else**.
HPI	The patient adds that he **has avoided most social contact** and that his art has suffered tremendously. He feels **debilitated** and wonders if he will ever emerge from his sadness.
Treatment	**Grief must be differentiated from major depression**, which has similar yet more severe and prolonged symptomatology. It is important that the physician explain the normal progression of mourning, provide reassurance, and validate the patient's pain.
Discussion	Pathologic grief is characterized by **intense or prolonged grief that causes functional or social impairment**, often for months. It is usually self-limited but can lead to or exacerbate chronic conditions such as depression, substance abuse, hypochondriasis, and organic disease. Distorted grief results when one aspect of grief, such as guilt, overshadows all others. Absent or delayed grief results from repression or denial of grief, which can subsequently lead to more prolonged or distorted grief.

ID/CC   A 26-year-old **female** presents with a sense of **bloating, swelling** of the limbs, headaches, **irritability, depression, and tension 4 days before her menses** are expected to begin.

HPI   She has **similar episodes almost every month**, each **beginning 4 to 5 days prior to her menses** and **ending shortly after her menstrual flow begins**.

Treatment   Making patients aware of the **cyclical nature** of premenstrual dysphoric disorder (PMDD) is a key part of treatment. Birth control pills (ORAL CONTRACEPTIVES) sometimes reduce the intensity of PMDD symptoms. Selective serotonin reuptake inhibitors (SSRIs) may be helpful, either continuously or in the luteal phase. Supportive psychotherapy may be beneficial.

Discussion   Studies indicate that 80% of women of reproductive age experience alterations of mood and/or physical discomfort before menses (premenstrual syndrome); however, only a relatively small number (3–5%) suffer affective symptoms severe enough to result in a psychiatric diagnosis of PMDD. Diagnosis requires that symptoms occur during the **luteal phase** and a symptom-free interval begins after onset of menstruation.

MOOD DISORDERS

PREMENSTRUAL DYSPHORIC DISORDER

ID/CC A 32-year-old male architect is in police custody for allegedly **exposing himself** and masturbating in front of a group of people in a subway station; he admits that he often feels an **overwhelming urge to expose himself** to people he does not know, adding that he becomes **aroused by the shock in their faces**.

HPI The patient is **ashamed of his actions** but claims that he **cannot resist his impulses**. He has been **arrested** on three previous occasions over the past 10 years, each time involving self-exposure to groups of women. The patient admits that he exposes himself often, especially when he is under emotional stress.

Treatment Counseling or group therapy may help. When possible, referral to a specialist is warranted. If patient tends to expose himself to children, physician must assess the possibility that he will become more active in his sexual involvement with them.

Discussion The diagnosis of exhibitionism rests on at least a **6-month history** of **recurrent sexual fantasies or acts** that involve the **exposure of one's genitals to strangers** and cause the **patient significant distress or impairment**. It tends to be a **chronic disorder that begins during adolescence** and may decrease in severity after age 40.

ID/CC   A 22-year-old male student claims that he **uses objects of women's clothing**, especially stockings and socks, to **become sexually aroused**; he frequently masturbates while rubbing such objects, which he has stolen from various women.

HPI   The patient **fears that he is "abnormal"** and that he will not be able to have a "regular" sex life because women will not understand his desires. He adds that he has **never had a sexual relationship or encounter**, although he is somewhat attracted to women. His medical history is unremarkable.

Treatment   If patient is distressed about condition, counseling or group therapy may help. When possible, referral to a specialist is warranted.

Discussion   The diagnosis of fetishism, a paraphilia, depends on at least a **6-month history** of **recurrent sexual fantasies or acts that involve inanimate objects** and that cause the patient significant distress or impairment. It tends to be a chronic disorder that **often begins during adolescence. Do not confuse with transvestic fetishism, which involves cross-dressing**.

ID/CC	A 31-year-old man reveals at the end of his annual physical that he has had **recurrent urges to rub against and fondle** the buttocks of women during his daily travels on the subway.
HPI	He has occasionally followed through on these desires but **feels guilty and embarrassed** about both his actions and thoughts. His personal report and a review of his medical chart reveal no significant medical or psychiatric history. The patient is single and not sexually active, which he attributes to his shy and inhibited behavior.
Treatment	Psychotherapy employing a cognitive-behavioral framework should focus heavily on specific paraphiliac behavior. Medroxyprogesterone acetate, a testosterone antagonist, can be used as a last resort to diminish sexual drive.
Discussion	Frotteurism is diagnosed if a patient has had, over the past **6 months, recurrent urges that involve rubbing against or touching a noncompliant person** and has **either acted on these impulses or become distressed by them**.

ID/CC	A 49-year-old **male** teacher is placed in police custody for allegedly **undressing and fondling** one of his **10-year-old** male students; upon questioning, he reveals that he is attracted only to boys in the third-grade age group and that he has an extensive **collection of pornographic images** of **children**.
HPI	The patient attempts to rationalize his behavior, saying that the boy enjoyed the experience and that it was "educational." He has long understood the social ramifications of his actions and states that he has tried many times to suppress his attractions, but to no avail. The patient denies being sexually attracted to women or adult men. His medical history is unremarkable.
Treatment	Counseling or group therapy may help. Referral to a specialist is warranted. Most states **require physicians to file reports of suspected sexual abuse of children immediately**.
Discussion	Pedophilia is the most common type of paraphilia. The diagnosis can be made with a **6-month history of sexual fantasies or acts that involve sexual activity with a prepubescent child**. Varying degrees of interaction may be involved, including undressing and observing the child; exposing oneself to the child; fondling; oral-genital contact; and anal or vaginal penetration with an object, finger, or penis. The physician must gauge the likelihood that a patient will act on his fantasies.

PEDOPHILIA

ID/CC A 32-year-old female is brought to the emergency department following a "fainting" episode; she claims that she developed dizziness and shortness of breath during sexual intercourse.

HPI Upon further questioning, she admits that her male partner, with her consent, routinely fastens a belt around her neck during intercourse, adding that she also submits routinely to being **bound, choked, and whipped** by her partner during sexual activity. She had "fantasies of being beaten and choked during sex" during adolescence but began to act on those fantasies only 2 years ago.

PE Patient alert and oriented and does not appear hypoxic; bruising around entire circumference of neck along with several horizontal scars on lower back.

Treatment If the patient is distressed about the condition, counseling or group therapy may help. Address the possible consequences of particular activities and assess the likelihood that the patient is being abused. When possible, refer to a specialist.

Discussion Sexual masochism is an example of a **paraphilia** that involves the **act of being made to suffer**. Such fantasies or acts cause the patient **significant distress, impairment, or injury**. Hypoxyphilia, in which one is oxygen-deprived by means of suffocation, strangling, or nitrate use, is a particularly dangerous form. Other forms include infantilism, physical bondage, sensory bondage (e.g., blindfolding), beating, cutting, electrical shocking, and humiliation. It tends to be a **chronic**, recurrent disorder that often begins during **early adulthood**.

ID/CC	A 30-year-old male is concerned about recurrent masturbatory **fantasies** in which he imagines himself **torturing and deriding various women**; he claims that he has never had such an encounter but that his fantasies are becoming more frequent and **violent** in nature.
HPI	The patient says that he has had such fantasies for as long as he can remember but adds that they have recently become more vivid and violent, causing him to fear that he is "sick" and that he may eventually hurt someone. He imagines himself exercising complete control over a victim by binding her and whipping her into submission. The patient has had "several" female sexual partners in the past and considers himself monogamous.
Treatment	Counseling, group therapy and aversive conditioning may help. The physician should assess the risk that such patients pose to others and take appropriate action. Referral to a specialist is warranted.
Discussion	Sexual sadism is an example of a **paraphilia** that involves **fantasies or acts** in which the **infliction of physical or emotional suffering is sexually arousing** to the patient. Such fantasies or acts cause the patient **significant distress or impairment**. Such acts may include humiliation, domination, physical bondage, sensory deprivation, beating, cutting, burning, electrical shocks, mutilation, rape, and killing. They may involve consenting or nonconsenting individuals. This tends to be a **chronic disorder that may begin in early childhood** and may become increasingly severe.

PARAPHILIA

SEXUAL SADISM

ID/CC	A 22-year-old **male** is brought to a physician for evaluation after **committing multiple crimes** and **attempting suicide**.
HPI	As a child he was hyperactive, did poorly in school, got into fights, abused animals, and was neglected by his drug-abusing parents. After dropping out of high school, he failed to hold down any job for an extended period of time and committed numerous crimes to support his drinking habit. He states that his suicide attempt was an impulsive act but adds that he **does not care what happens to him or anyone else**. He **feels no remorse** for the pain he has inflicted on others.
PE	Numerous scars from fights and accidents.
Treatment	Inpatient psychotherapy with confrontation and group therapy are treatment of choice.
Discussion	Antisocial personality disorder is characterized by an **inability to conform to social norms** as well as by **repetitive criminal behavior**. Males are four times more likely to be affected than females.

ID/CC   A 23-year-old male complains of having too few friends and an **unreasonable fear of new experiences**.

HPI   He reports that his **shyness** has frequently prevented him from participating in social activities. At times, his fear of criticism has affected his performance in school.

Treatment   Group therapy can help.

Discussion   People with avoidant personality disorder often have social phobia as well. They are **sensitive to rejection, socially withdrawn, and shy**. Avoidant personality disorder can be differentiated from schizoid personality disorder in that schizoid individuals are happy being alone, whereas avoidant individuals are **distressed at the prospect of being alone**.

AVOIDANT PERSONALITY DISORDER

ID/CC	During a routine physical exam, a young female patient tells her physician that she has **fallen in love with him**; when he recommends that she see another physician, she **threatens to commit suicide**.
HPI	She denies any depression or suicidal ideation in the past.
Treatment	Psychiatric consultation and behavioral psychotherapy can be effective over time.
Discussion	Characteristics of such a personality disorder include **unstable mood and behavior, suicide attempts, boredom, splitting, feelings of emptiness and loneliness**, and **impulsiveness**.

BORDERLINE PERSONALITY DISORDER

ID/CC   A 49-year-old female homemaker complains of disillusionment with her marriage and general sadness; she states that she **feels insecure when left on her own** and has great **difficulty asserting herself**.

HPI   She adds that she considers herself a **"follower"** who has always **left all decision making to her husband**. She describes her husband as an intense and domineering man who makes many demands. She has few friends other than the acquaintances she has met through her husband.

Treatment   Counseling and group therapy may help. Training in assertiveness and in developing social skills may also be of value.

Discussion   Dependent personality disorder denotes a **chronic, excessive dependence on others**. Such patients frequently **defer decision making** to others, **tolerate mistreatment, place others' needs before their own**, and have **difficulty being assertive**. Patients may also demonstrate **low self-esteem, insecurity**, and a **longing to be in a relationship**.

DEPENDENT PERSONALITY DISORDER

ID/CC	A 27-year-old, **charming, scantily clad woman** complains of suicidal feelings and **vague musculoskeletal pain**; she asks to see "the best doctor in the hospital."
HPI	She explains how she is **annoyed by a coworker who has become the center of attention at the office**. The patient **behaves seductively** and exhibits inappropriately **dramatic emotions** while omitting important details in her responses. She has a history of multiple suicide attempts, after which she claims to have **received sympathy from a multitude of "close friends."**
PE	Small, shallow scars on wrists from past suicide attempts.
Treatment	Patients with minor impairment can be treated with psychotherapy.
Discussion	Histrionic personality disorder has a 2% prevalence in the overall population and has significant comorbidity with depression, substance abuse, and somatization disorder. People suffering from this personality disorder are **dramatic, extroverted, and emotional; exhibit sexually provocative behavior**; and are unable to maintain intimate relationships (although they often **overstate the closeness of their friendships**). These patients are often fundamentally insecure, and their theatrics are generally efforts to obtain love, support, and reassurance. Cluster B personality disorder.

ID/CC A 45-year-old man is admitted to the medical unit following a heart attack; a psych consult is requested when nurses report that his **offensive behavior** is disrupting the staff and other patients.

HPI When questioned, the patient is dismissive and prefers instead to discuss his "beautiful girlfriend," new sports car, and **widespread influence**. He denies having had a heart attack and claims that it was just "minor heartburn." He loudly belittles the staff for being inattentive and claims that the consulting physician is "the only one here who can appreciate me."

Labs ECG and labs consistent with diagnosis of myocardial infarction.

Treatment Patients benefit from psychotherapy but must be **treated with sensitivity and empathy, as confronting these difficult issues may be perceived as humiliating**.

Discussion Patients with narcissistic personality disorder will often **ignore or deny illness** to protect their fragile self-esteem. These patients often have a **poor sense of self**; they compensate by **soliciting attention and praise** from others and by creating an **image of power, wealth, and attractiveness**. They often **lack empathy and exhibit a strong sense of entitlement**. They cope best with a medical setting in which they feel appreciated and admired. Cluster B personality disorder.

NARCISSISTIC PERSONALITY DISORDER

ID/CC   A 34-year-old **male** complains of anxiety over not doing his work well enough along with an inability to enjoy recreational activities that he himself has organized.

HPI   He describes **making lists and protocols**, and he remarks about how well he is able to organize activities. He has few friends because **work occupies most of his time**. He tends to be very thrifty and **adheres rigidly to moral and ethical values**. People often find it difficult to work with him because he is slow and **meticulous** and **demands perfection** of his coworkers.

Treatment   Long-term psychotherapy is of benefit.

Discussion   Obsessive-compulsive personality disorder affects males twice as often as females. Cluster C personality disorder.

OBSESSIVE-COMPULSIVE PERSONALITY DISORDER

ID/CC	A 55-year-old male **insists that his physician has deliberately prescribed harmful drugs for him** and states that he will file a malpractice suit against the doctor.
HPI	The patient is **hostile** and angry.
PE	Physical examination normal, although patient is suspicious and guarded.
Treatment	Patients may benefit from supportive therapy. Medical management should include clear explanations of procedures and medications.
Discussion	A patient with paranoid personality disorder is characteristically **suspicious and mistrustful, interpreting the motives of others as malevolent**. He often holds others responsible for his problems. Cluster A personality disorder.

PARANOID PERSONALITY DISORDER

ID/CC   A 48-year-old obese diabetic woman consults a physician for help in dieting, after which the doctor prepares a diet for her and discusses it with her in detail.

HPI   The patient **misses her next two follow-up appointments** and does not return calls from the office staff. She eventually returns for another visit but is **30 minutes late**. She has **gained some weight** but claims that she has followed the diet regimen.

Treatment   **Insight-oriented therapy** may help these patients express anger and frustration in a more direct manner. Physicians should try to involve such patients more actively in planning their medical treatment.

Discussion   Characteristics of passive-aggressive personality disorder include **procrastination, stubbornness, inefficiency, and passive resistance to authority and responsibility**. This disorder is no longer recognized in DSM-IV.

ID/CC	A 40-year-old **scientist** presents for a work physical, where questioning reveals that he has **no contact with his family, does not maintain any friendships**, and lives alone.
HPI	The patient **seems apathetic** with regard to his apparent dearth of social support structures. He has **never engaged in dating or other social activities**. He prefers to work alone at home and **cannot name any hobbies or activities that he finds enjoyable**.
Treatment	Behavioral therapy targeting social integration may be useful.
Discussion	**A lifelong pattern of voluntary social withdrawal without psychosis** is characteristic of patients suffering from schizoid personality disorder. Cluster A personality disorder.

SCHIZOID PERSONALITY DISORDER

ID/CC   A 38-year-old woman presents to a local clinic complaining that her left hand has disappeared.

HPI   The patient is wearing **mismatched shoes** and has **colored her eyebrows with red lipstick**. When the physician examines her hands, she suddenly seems relieved and thanks him for restoring her missing hand. The patient lives alone and reports that she **avoids family and neighbors because they "can't be trusted."** She also claims that she can read others' minds.

PE   Inappropriate affect; odd appearance; no hallucinations or delusions.

Treatment   Low-dose neuroleptics may alleviate the social anxiety, peculiar thought patterns, and perceptual illusions of schizotypal patients. Supportive therapy can be used to encourage patients to become involved in more social activities.

Discussion   Schizotypal personality disorder is characterized by a **peculiar appearance and odd thought patterns** and behavior in the **absence of psychosis**. These patients tend to become **socially isolated**. Cluster A personality disorder.

ID/CC	A 40-year-old female high-school teacher is brought to the ER by her colleagues because they are alarmed by her odd behavior.
HPI	Her coworkers noticed that she has become increasingly **anxious** of late and has begun to talk about people who are allegedly **watching her behind her back**. Her husband adds that she recently refused to get ready for bed and began pacing around the room looking in the closet and under the bed for people hiding there.
PE	Patient **anxious and delusional** on mental status exam.
Labs	No evidence of drug abuse on urinary screen.
Treatment	Hospitalization is recommended, with an antipsychotic medication given for the acute episode.

BRIEF PSYCHOTIC EPISODE

ID/CC	A 35-year-old male tells his doctor that people at work hate him and have **conspired to eliminate him** because he complained about them to management 10 years ago.
HPI	The patient's behavior and speech are normal. He denies any depression or suicidal ideation. His wife tells the physician that aside from his beliefs regarding his coworkers, he **participates normally in family activities**.
PE	Neurologic exam normal; higher mental functions normal; **belief unshakable**.
Treatment	Psychotherapy and antipsychotic medication can be beneficial, but delusional disorders are often refractory to treatment (vs. schizophrenia).
Discussion	Delusions are **fixed and culturally inappropriate but nonbizarre beliefs** that a patient holds **despite all reasonable evidence to the contrary**. Individuals with delusional disorder have one fixed delusional system but are **otherwise relatively functional** (vs. schizophrenics).

A 73-year-old male is transferred to the ICU immediately following hip replacement surgery; on his second day in the unit, he **attempts to rise from bed** to escape the **"faces flying over his bed."**

HPI The nurse in charge of his care reports that he has become **progressively disoriented** and has **not slept well** since his admission to the unit. He has no history of dementia.

Treatment Haloperidol, a neuroleptic, should be given as a sedative. Lorazepam can be used, although benzodiazepines may cause anterograde amnesia and may exacerbate disinhibited behavior. Treatment of underlying medical condition causing the patient's mental status change is essential.

Discussion The **disorienting environment of the hospital** often makes patients susceptible to hospital-induced psychosis or delirium.

ICU PSYCHOSIS

PSYCHOTIC DISORDERS

ID/CC   A **20-year-old man** is brought into the ER after he was discovered trying to hang himself.

HPI   The patient has become quiet and **withdrawn**, avoiding social activities and school events. His roommate reports that for the **past 6 months**, many friends have commented on his increasingly **peculiar behavior**. The roommate also reports that 2 months ago the patient began **mumbling to himself** and often pausing as if he were **listening to someone else**. Upon psychiatric evaluation, the patient **speaks in a disorganized fashion** and complains that a **voice told him to kill himself**. Further questioning reveals that the patient is still hearing the voice, which maintains a **running commentary of derisive remarks** regarding the patient's personality and actions.

Labs   Drug screen negative (ruling out drug-induced psychosis).

Imaging   MR, brain: normal or mild atrophy.

Treatment   Neuroleptic agents can be used to control psychotic symptoms. Combining benzodiazepines with neuroleptics may be appropriate in acute situations. Hospitalization may be necessary. Long-term supportive psychotherapy along with pharmacotherapy should be utilized.

Discussion   Acute schizophrenia has a 1% prevalence, with onset usually occurring in the **early 20s to 30s**. Current research suggests that schizophrenia is due to a **defect in the dopaminergic** system. Neuroleptics can cause a variety of side effects, including anticholinergic effects, postural hypertension, and tardive dyskinesia.

SCHIZOPHRENIA—ACUTE

ID/CC A 22-year-old woman is brought to the psych ER by the police after she was found loitering in a large shopping mall; she is not responsive to questioning aside from an occasional parrot-like echoing of the interviewer's words.

HPI She is **unkempt**, dirty, and wearing shorts despite near-freezing temperatures. Her mother, with whom she lives, reports that within the past 2 years the patient has become increasingly "sullen" and has periods during which she **"refuses to speak or even budge."** The mother has also noticed that the patient often speaks in a loose, tangential fashion. The mother complains that she is too busy to pay attention to her daughter's problems but nonetheless claims that her daughter is just "going through a phase." The patient recently withdrew from her classes at the local college.

PE **Posture fairly rigid** throughout examination; patient's limbs maintain various positions induced by physician during exam (WAXY FLEXIBILITY OR CATALEPSY).

Labs Drug/EtOH screen negative.

Treatment Treat schizophrenia; patients should also be carefully monitored to prevent self-injury or malnutrition.

Discussion Patients with catatonic schizophrenia may exhibit peculiar voluntary movements, grimacing, senseless repetition of words spoken by another (ECHOLALIA), and repetitive imitation of another person's movements (ECHOPRAXIA). General medical disorders, substance abuse, and major depression must be ruled out.

SCHIZOPHRENIA—CATATONIC

ID/CC   A thin, **poorly groomed 25-year-old man** is brought to the ER by a concerned neighbor who claims that the patient stopped going to work 3 weeks ago and often speaks in a **nonsensical, discontinuous fashion**; she strongly suspects alcohol abuse but can find no evidence of it in his household.

HPI   The neighbor also states that within the past year the patient has exhibited **increasingly "bizarre" behavior**, such as failing to wash himself, maintain his appearance, or eat properly. Once friendly and talkative, the patient now avoids other people and spends hours cutting shapes out of the newspaper. The patient attempts to answer the physician's questions but is quickly sidetracked, frequently lapsing into **silence or incoherence**. His **speech is difficult to follow** and is often punctuated by laughing or giggling that is seemingly unrelated to the subject at hand.

Labs   Drug/EtOH screen negative.

Treatment   As with other types of schizophrenia, this patient may respond to neuroleptic medications combined with long-term supportive psychotherapy.

Discussion   Patients with the disorganized subtype of schizophrenia exhibit **disorganized speech, disorganized behavior, and flat/ inappropriate affect**. Their lack of goal orientation may affect their ability to perform activities of daily living.

ID/CC A 17-year-old man is brought by his parents to the psych ER because they have been increasingly alarmed by his **suspicious** and unpredictable demeanor over the past 6 months.

HPI The patient reveals to the interviewing psychiatrist that he believes his parents are **trying to kill him**. He also explains that he read an article in the local paper which he has interpreted to mean that somebody is trying **to warn him of the danger**. His teachers have observed that the patient has become much more **withdrawn** and socializes less frequently with his classmates.

Labs Drug/EtOH screen negative.

Treatment As with other types of schizophrenia, this patient may respond to neuroleptic medications combined with long-term supportive psychotherapy.

Discussion Despite treatment with neuroleptics and supportive psychotherapy, patients with paranoid schizophrenia may never regain their former level of functioning.

ID/CC A 35-year-old woman with an extensive psychiatric history comes to her internist's office wearing three large skirts layered over a pair of pants despite the mild summer weather; she denies having hallucinations or hearing voices but explains that her deceased mother warned her to dress warmly.

HPI The patient **speaks in a loose, tangential fashion and occasionally lapses into incoherent speech.** She has been hospitalized six times for inability to care for herself and acute psychosis. During these episodes, she experienced vivid visual hallucinations involving various deceased family members and expressed the belief that those family members wanted to kill her. **Her last hospitalization was 3 years ago.**

Labs Drug/EtOH screen negative.

Treatment Neuroleptics, antidepressants, and supportive psychotherapy.

Discussion The diagnosis of residual-type schizophrenia can be made if **negative symptoms are still present or if patients present with two positive symptoms (delusions, hallucinations, disorganized speech, or grossly disorganized/catatonic behavior) in attenuated form.**

ID/CC   A 29-year-old woman presents for a follow-up visit following a 3-week **remission from a 4-month period of psychotic episodes**.

HPI   During that 4-month period, the patient **heard voices** conversing with one another and suspected that her mind **was being controlled by a voice on the radio**. These auditory hallucinations were much more intrusive in the morning. The patient attempted to drown out the voices by listening to a Walkman and managed to maintain marginal performance at her nighttime cleaning job. At the time of this visit, the patient denies hearing any voices and no longer holds the delusion of mind control, reporting that her performance at work has improved significantly.

Labs   Lab studies normal.

Treatment   During the symptomatic period, the patient may have responded to neuroleptic medications.

Discussion   The diagnosis of schizophreniform disorder is based on **schizophrenia-like symptoms for more than 1 month but less than 6 months**. If the patient is symptomatic but has been so for less than 6 months, the diagnosis should be "schizophreniform—provisional." One-third of these patients recover within 6 months; the remainder progress to a diagnosis of schizophrenia.

SCHIZOPHRENIFORM DISORDER

ID/CC A 52-year-old female accountant complains that she has had **difficulty falling and staying asleep** for 2 months; she states that the sleep she does manage to get is **not restful** and that she is easily awakened by noises.

HPI The patient adds that she is **fatigued during the day** and as a result is performing poorly at her job. She says that she has always been a "light" sleeper. She denies feeling depressed, although she admits that she gets irritable when tired. She takes no medications and drinks two cups of coffee each day, always before noon.

PE The patient appears fatigued but is otherwise in good health.

Treatment **Rule out other potentially precipitating disorders, especially depression. Institute sleep hygiene measures**, e.g., sleep only as much as is necessary; establish regular hours for sleep; exercise; avoid caffeine, alcohol, tobacco, and other stimulants; leave the bed when not tired. Hypnotic agents (e.g., benzodiazepines) may aid in short-term management.

Discussion Complaints of insomnia are most prevalent among women and the elderly. Younger patients tend to report more difficulty in initiating sleep, while the elderly tend to have more difficulty maintaining sleep. A diagnosis of primary insomnia depends on excluding other causes. Differential diagnosis includes circadian rhythm disorder, primary hypersomnia, narcolepsy, sleep apnea, parasomnias, and sleep disorders secondary to other medical and psychiatric disorders.

ID/CC   A **12-year-old girl** is brought to her pediatrician by her parents, who report that she has been repeatedly **walking "like a zombie" in her sleep**. Twice she has walked into the closet and urinated there in her sleep.

HPI   It is **difficult to awaken** the patient during these episodes, and she is **only briefly confused minutes upon awakening and does not recall the episode.** Her parents are very concerned about her inappropriate behavior and fear for her safety. Her mother adds that the patient has **begun to avoid her classmates' slumber parties** and is **reluctant to stay with relatives overnight**. They fear that she is becoming **socially isolated as a result**. The patient has no history of seizures or similar episodes during the day.

PE   Physical exam normal; mental status exam unremarkable; some anxiety noted.

Treatment   Parents should be reassured that sleepwalking usually disappears spontaneously during early adolescence. Sharp objects and obstacles should be removed from the floor. A course of short-acting barbiturates may be useful in conjunction with psychotherapy.

Discussion   Somnambulism occurs in delta sleep, usually during the first third of the night. Sleepwalking disorder in adults warrants psychiatric evaluation. Post-traumatic stress disorder, acute stress disorder, and somatoform disorder should be part of the differential.

SLEEPWALKING DISORDER

ID/CC	A **17-year-old woman** in her first year of college presents to the student health services with complaints of fever and sore throat.
HPI	Careful questioning reveals that the patient is not physically ill but rather made up the story out of reluctance to admit her desire to see if "someone can do something about my lips." She states that her **lips "are too fat"** and that their appearance **impedes her ability to socialize normally** with her peers. Her embarrassment has progressed to such a degree that she no longer attends her classes.
PE	Physical exam reveals a healthy and attractive young woman.
Treatment	Psychiatric intervention using group or individual therapy and focusing on psychosocial functions and body image has proven effective. Pharmacologic therapy using antidepressants or antipsychotics has shown less success.
Discussion	Body dysmorphic disorder is **characterized by a preoccupation with an imagined defect in appearance that causes clinically significant distress or impairment in social, occupational, or other important areas of functioning** and excludes any other mental disorder. Some researchers regard this syndrome as a prodrome of schizophrenia.

BODY DYSMORPHIC DISORDER

ID/CC   A 26-year-old female is brought to her family physician with complaints of an **inability to speak or to move** the right side of body for the past hour.

HPI   She **received news of the death** of her 3-year-old child **immediately before the onset of her symptoms**. Her previous history, as elicited from her spouse, suggests an **underlying dependent personality disorder**. She comes from a rural background and is not well educated.

PE   **Fundus, pupils, deep tendon reflexes normal**; mutism noted; **"la belle indifférence"** to symptoms.

Treatment   Psychotherapy used to detect underlying conflict and repressed thoughts; emotional release sought through hypnosis.

Discussion   Conversion disorder is a **type of somatoform disorder**.

CONVERSION DISORDER

ID/CC	A 23-year-old medical student complains of abdominal pain that has lasted for over 6 months.
HPI	The patient **believes that his abdominal pain is indicative of a serious illness**. Although previous medical examinations by several other physicians found **no serious pathology**, he continues to believe that he has a severe medical problem. **His preoccupation with the "disease"** has begun to interfere with his social and occupational activities.
PE	Poorly localized abdominal tenderness.
Labs	Routine laboratory studies normal.
Treatment	Telling the patient that no pathology exists is often futile; best results are achieved by helping patient cope with perceived illness.
Discussion	Hypochondriasis must be differentiated from somatization disorders, anxiety disorders, and depressive disorders. If any of these disorders is present, treatment of the underlying condition will often lead to the resolution of hypochondriasis.

HYPOCHONDRIASIS

ID/CC	A 30-year-old **male** complains of **persistent inability to maintain an erection during intercourse**.
HPI	He states that his disorder is causing difficulty in his marriage. He has no history of psychiatric disorder and **denies any drug or medication use**. He has no acute or chronic illness and no history of genitourinary surgery.
PE	VS: BP normal.
Labs	Lytes: normal. Testosterone, TSH, LH, FSH, and prolactin normal; **nocturnal penile tumescence reveals erection** during REM sleep.
Treatment	**Individual and couples therapy is treatment of choice**. If a medication can be implicated, it should be changed.
Discussion	Almost **90%** of male erectile dysfunction is believed to be of **psychogenic origin**. Medication- and acute illness-induced erectile dysfunction can also occur. Substances known to cause erectile dysfunction include some tricyclic antidepressants, MAO inhibitors, anticholinergics, ethanol, and amphetamines. Disorders of the hypothalamic-pituitary axis, thyroid, and kidneys must be ruled out.

MALE ERECTILE DISORDER—PSYCHOGENIC

ID/CC   A 29-year-old woman presents to her family physician following a **positive home-pregnancy test**.

HPI   She reports an 8-week history of amenorrhea accompanied by breast tenderness, malaise, lassitude, and nausea. A repeat **pregnancy test in the doctor's office is positive for hCG**. The patient is elated because she has been trying to become pregnant for 1 year.

PE   Weight gain of 4 pounds in 6 weeks; uterus soft and enlarged; cervix soft and cyanotic.

Imaging   US, uterus: at week 13 shows **empty uterine cavity without any evidence of fetal parts or gestational sac**; no evidence of ectopic pregnancy.

Discussion False pregnancy (PSEUDOCYESIS) can manifest with many of the physical signs and symptoms of pregnancy. It may occur in women who have a strong desire to be pregnant or in women with a strong fear of pregnancy.

PSEUDOCYESIS

ID/CC   A 36-year-old **woman** presents to the ER with a 2-day history of progressive right lower quadrant pain.

HPI   A review of systems reveals **numerous symptoms**. Further questioning reveals that she has been sickly since **early adolescence** with numerous chronic symptoms, including **nausea, bloating, polyarticular joint pain, dyspareunia, dysmenorrhea, and difficulty swallowing**. She is **frustrated with her many ailments** and by **her failure to find a medical explanation for them** despite visits to numerous physicians. The patient also reveals that she has been feeling "very stressed out" due to an impending divorce and her mother's recent death.

PE   **Physical exam reveals no abnormalities**.

Labs   No leukocytosis.

Treatment   Treatment should include employment of therapeutic alliance, scheduling of regular appointments, and crisis intervention utilizing psychiatric consult services. Prognostic outlook is fair. These individuals are often highly resistant to psychiatric referral.

Discussion   Differential diagnosis includes physical disease and depression. The onset of somatization disorder occurs before age 30. Almost 1% of all women are affected. There is a 20% concordance rate for first-degree female relatives. Symptoms **are not intentionally feigned** or produced (vs. factitious disorder).

SOMATIZATION DISORDER

ID/CC A 20-year-old female complains of **severe pain** that **prevents her from attaining the social and occupational goals** she has set for herself.

HPI The patient receives temporary relief with physical therapy, but the pain inevitably returns some time later. **Stress tends to exacerbate the pain**.

PE The pain does not follow any anatomic distribution.

Labs Physical examination normal.

Treatment Counseling with goal of improving coping strategies is primary treatment; judicious use of antidepressants and anxiolytics may also help.

Discussion Confronting patients with somatoform disorder may worsen symptoms.

ID/CC   A 27-year-old woman presenting for her annual gynecologic exam reveals that she has been unable to participate in sexual intercourse because of **severe vaginal contractions** elicited by attempts at penile penetration of the vagina.

HPI   Further questioning reveals that the patient has experienced these symptoms many times in the past with various sexual partners. She has been dating her current partner for 4 months and has become progressively anxious with respect to their heightened sexual activity; **she wishes to have intercourse** with him yet fears a repetition of past failures. She also reports difficulty in inserting tampons.

PE   Genital examination incomplete because of **inability to insert speculum**.

Treatment   Successful treatment is based in behavioral methods that desensitize patient to experience of penetration.

Discussion   The contractions are **involuntary reflex spasms of the muscles of the vagina**. Vaginismus is **sometimes secondary to genital/ sexual trauma**.

VAGINISMUS

ID/CC   A successful 50-year-old business executive becomes **agitated** upon his admission to an orthopedic ward with a fractured femur; **he complains that people are making derogatory comments about him** and are accusing him of impotence (PARANOID DELUSIONS).

HPI   On persistent questioning, he admits to **"moderate" alcohol intake**. There is no personal, past, or family history suggestive of any major psychiatric illness.

PE   Psychomotor **agitation; anxious** and slightly tremulous but well oriented; remainder of neurologic, funduscopic, and systemic exam normal.

Treatment   **Haloperidol** is effective in relieving hallucinosis.

Discussion   **Auditory hallucinations** and/or **paranoid delusions** can occur with **alcohol withdrawal**, as can **anxiety** and **sadness**. Assessment of alcohol intake is an important part of the differential in any patient presenting with these symptoms.

ALCOHOLIC HALLUCINOSIS

ID/CC A 20-year-old male is brought to the emergency room in a severely **agitated** state.

HPI According to a friend, the patient **took "angel dust"** about an hour before his arrival in the ER.

PE Patient severely agitated, **belligerent**, emotionally **labile**, and **frightened; speech slurred** (DYSARTHRIA); vertical and **horizontal nystagmus** noted. Diminished response to painful stimuli.

Labs UA: **phencyclidine (PCP) metabolites**.

Treatment **Diazepam and minimizing sensory stimulation** are useful in controlling agitated state.

Discussion PCP can induce a psychosis similar to schizophrenia.

PCP INTOXICATION

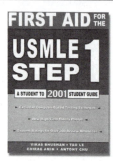
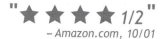
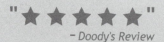
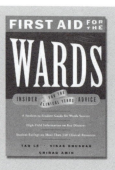
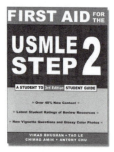
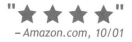
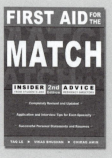